THE GOLDMAN GUIDE TO PSYCHIATRY

with
DSM-5 Update

David Eckstein Goldman, JD, DO, FCLM, FAPA
Physician/Psychiatrist/Attorney At Law

The Goldman Guide to Psychiatry
with DSM-5 Update

David Eckstein Goldman, JD, DO, FCLM, FAPA
Physician/Psychiatrist/Attorney At Law

Published by:
Miracle Press
P. O. Box 765
Jacksonville, Illinois 62651

www.thegoldmangroup.org

Cover design and interior layout: www.TheBookProducer.com
Printed in the United States of America

ISBN 978-0-9774185-4-1

I want to dedicate this book to my parents and brother thanking them for all their guidance, love, support, and for always being there.

CONTENTS

ABOUT THE AUTHOR

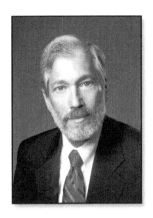

Dr. Goldman graduated from the University of Illinois in Champaign-Urbana, Illinois, in 1973, having received his Bachelor of Arts Degree with a major in History, a focus in Religious Studies, and a double minor in Psychology and Sociology.

After completing his undergraduate studies, Dr. Goldman attended Washington University School of Law, receiving his Juris Doctorate Degree in 1976. From 1976 until beginning medical school in 1987, he served as secretary-treasurer and corporate legal counsel for Central Industries, Inc.

In 1987, Dr. Goldman entered medical school at the Kirksville College of Osteopathic Medicine, graduating in 1991 with his Doctor of Osteopathy degree. He completed a traditional transitional rotating internship at the Kirksville Osteopathic Medical Center in Kirksville, Missouri, in 1992, after which time he began his residency training in Psychiatry at Vanderbilt University Medical Center in Nashville, Tennessee. Dr. Goldman completed his residency training in 1996, and completed his Fellowship training in Child and Adolescent Psychiatry in 1997, also at Vanderbilt University Medical Center.

After completing his Residency and Fellowship training, Dr. Goldman returned to Springfield, Illinois, establishing his practice in psychiatry. He is the Medical Director for The Goldman Group, LLC. and serves as a medicolegal consultant, as well as continuing his private psychotherapy and psychopharmacology management practice. He also serves as a professor at both Southern Illinois University Medical School in Springfield, Illinois, and at the Kirksville College of Osteopathic Medicine in Kirksville, Missouri.

Dr. Goldman was the 2001 and the 2011 recipient of the Max Gutensohn *Professor of the Year Award* at ATSU/Kirksville College of Osteopathic Medicine. In 2001 Dr. Goldman was awarded the *Order of Merlin Shield* by the International Brotherhood of Magicians and in 2016 he was awarded the *Order of Merlin Excalibur* by the International Brotherhood of Magicians. In 2007, he was one of 18 psychiatrists selected from among the nation's physicians to receive the NAMI *Exemplary Psychiatrist Award* presented at the international meeting of the American Psychiatric Association. Dr. Goldman was elected to Fellowship in the American Psychiatric Association in 2015.

The Triad of Psychiatry

Sigmund Freud, considered the father of psychoanalysis and modern psychiatry, provided 2 approaches to conceptualizing the human mind: the structural schema and the topographic schema (see Chapter 13). Adding a diagnostic schema (Table) provides the clinician an overview of the major psychiatric disorders.

Freud's Structural Schema	*Freud's Topographic Schema*	*Goldman's Diagnostic Schema*
• Id • Ego • Superego	• Conscious • Preconscious • Unconscious	• Mood Disorder • Anxiety Disorder • Thought Disorder

Table. Goldman's Diagnostic Schema

Affective/Mood Disorder	Anxiety Disorder	Thought Disorder
Adjustment disorder	Panic disorder (with or without agoraphobia)	Brief reactive psychosis
Major depressive disorder (with or without psychotic features)	Generalized anxiety disorder	Schizophreniform disorder
Dysthymic disorder	Specific phobia	Schizophrenia
Cyclothymic disorder	Social phobia	
Bipolar disorder	Acute stress disorder/post-traumatic stress disorder	
	Obsessive-compulsive disorder - - - - - - - - ➔	Delusional disorder

Affective/Mood Disorder　　　　　　　　　　　　　　**Thought Disorder**
↑ - - - - - - - - - - - - - Schizoaffective Disorder - - - - - - - - - - - - - ↑

Goldman's Diagnostic Schema illustrates the overarching construct of psychiatry divided into the disorders of mood, anxiety, and thought. These 3 separate categories sometimes become blurred. A mood disorder is often intertwined with anxiety; an anxiety disorder often begets a mood disorder. A mood disorder can become so severe that thought processes become disorganized, as in major depressive disorder with psychotic features. Obsessive-compulsive disorder can become so overwhelming and entrenched that it can look and feel like a delusional disorder, a form of thought disorder.

Diagnoses are not always clearly discrete. The above-listed categories of mood, anxiety, and thought intersect and interweave. While many psychiatric diagnoses fall outside the confines of the categories of mood, anxiety, and thought, it is these 3 categories that constitute the overarching construct of psychiatry. The purpose of this book is to assist in understanding and simplifying the complexities of the diagnoses and to facilitate treatment approaches.

CHAPTER ONE

Recognition and Treatment of Mood Disorders

Mood disorders are best considered in a progression from the least severe of conditions to the most disruptive of conditions. Euthymia is the baseline that equates to balanced mood, and mood disorders are disruptions above and below this balance. Psychiatry assesses the descents and elevations in mood (Figure 1).

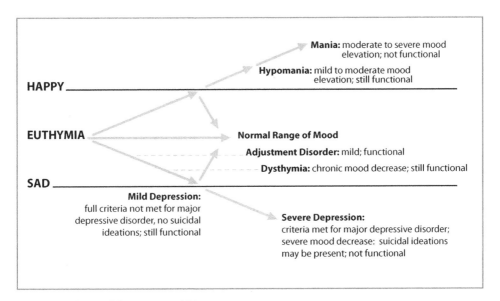

Figure 1. The Goldman Mood Map

TYPES OF MOOD DISORDERS

Moods Below Euthymia

Adjustment Disorder. Externalized psychosocial stressors, such as failing an examination, losing a job, experiencing a divorce, or losing a loved one, can disrupt life outlook. Individuals may experience difficulty in adjusting to these occurrences and their results. An adjustment disorder involves a readily identifiable psychosocial stressor occurring within 3 months of the decline in life outlook. Typically, return to baseline functioning should occur within 6 months of resolution of the life event. The adjustment disorder can last longer than 6 months, however, if it is a response to a chronic stressor or one with continuing consequences. An adjustment disorder is milder than a major depressive disorder. Individuals with an adjustment disorder typically remain functional in their daily lives, yet recognize the need for help.

Dysthymic Disorder (Dysthymia). Presenting as a long-term mild-to-moderate decline in mood, dysthymia manifests in adults as a chronic decreased mood lasting for most of the day, every day, for 2 years or more. In children or adolescents, the diagnosis should be suspected if 1 year of chronic decreased mood or irritability has occurred. Along with decreased mood, 2 of the following must also be present:

- Change in appetite
- Change in sleep patterns
- Decrease in concentration or memory
- Decrease in energy
- Decrease in self-esteem
- Feelings of hopelessness

Dysthymia is hallmarked by a loss of interest in life activities and decreased mood that does not meet the criteria for a major depressive disorder. It presents as a milder form of chronic depression. Unfortunately, while its day-to-day symptomatology may not be as severe as that found in major depressive disorder, because of its long-term chronicity, it can have more devastating results in someone's social and occupational life. Individuals suffering from dysthymia may experience episodes of major depressive disorder as well. When these individuals suffer superimposed episodes of major depression, it is termed *double depression*. To make this diagnosis, there cannot be an absence of the symptoms for more than 2 consecutive months (during the 2 year period for adults/1 year period for children).

Major Depressive Disorder. **The hallmark of major depressive disorder is the major depressive episode.** Individuals suffering a major depressive episode experience at least 5 of 9 of the below listed symptoms as disruptions in their lives most of the day, every day, for 2 consecutive weeks:

- Changes in motor functioning (either agitation or retardation)
- Changes in sleep patterns (either increased or decreased sleep)
- Changes in weight (either weight loss or gain)
- Depressed mood
- Disturbance in the ability to concentrate or remember things
- Feelings of worthlessness, guilt, or shame
- Loss of daily energy
- Loss of interest in life activities
- Thoughts of dying, including suicidal thoughts

To meet the criteria of a major depressive episode, at least one of the life disruptions must be either loss of interest in life activities (anhedonia) or a depressed mood. The impact of the combination of the disturbances leaves the individual marginally functional at best, nonfunctioning at worst.

Moods Above Euthymia

Bipolar Disorder. The disease of bipolar disorder is comprised of either a manic episode with or without a depressive episode, or a hypomanic episode with one or recurrent depressive episodes. Hypomania and mania are the hallmark components for diagnosing bipolar disorder, differentiating it from a unipolar depression which is limited to mood below euthymia.

Hypomanic and Manic Episodes. Hypomania involves either mild-to-moderate elevation of mood or irritability. Individuals with a mildly or moderately elevated or irritable mood lasting at least 4 days who concurrently experience at least 3 (4 if irritable) of the behaviors listed below are having a hypomanic episode. If the elevated mood or irritability lasts a week or more along with the additional symptoms, the person should be diagnosed as having a manic episode:

- Subjective feeling of racing thoughts
- Disturbance in concentration and focus
- Inappropriately elevated self-esteem
- Uncharacteristic risk-taking behavior
- Increase in motor activity
- Increase in pursuing goals and tasks
- Increase in talkativeness
- Less need for sleep

THE DIAGNOSIS AND TREATMENT OF DEPRESSION

Diagnosing Depression

In major depressive disorder, there is disturbance in the individual's SAMCEL(S) (Box 1) all day, every day for at least 2 weeks. There are 2 types of depression, typical depression, affecting 52% to 58% of depressed individuals; and atypical depression, affecting 42% to 48% of depressed individuals.

Utilizing SAMCEL(S) provides the data to differentiate between the 2 types of depressive disorder. The individual is asked a series of questions as follows:

- How is your sleep? Do you have any difficulty in:
  - ❑ Initiating sleep?
  - ❑ Maintaining sleep?
  - ❑ Awakening/not feeling rested on awakening?
- How is your appetite?
  - ❑ Increased?
  - ❑ Decreased?
  - ❑ The same as usual?
- How is your memory?
  - ❑ Increased?
  - ❑ Decreased?
  - ❑ The same as usual?
- How is your concentration?
  - ❑ Increased?
  - ❑ Decreased?
  - ❑ The same as usual?
- How is your energy?
  - ❑ Increased?
  - ❑ Decreased?
  - ❑ The same as usual?
- How is your libido (interest in sexual activity)?
  - ❑ Increased?
  - ❑ Decreased?
  - ❑ The same as usual?
- Are you having any suicidal thoughts? Do you
  - ❑ Want to hurt yourself?
  - ❑ Want to kill yourself?
  - ❑ Want to die?

Box 1. SAMCEL(S) the Psychiatric Vital Signs

In other medical specialties, the individual's baseline state of health is reflected in the vital signs of blood pressure, body temperature, and heart rate. In psychiatry, 6 neurovegetative functioning inventory indices represent the individual's psychiatric vital signs and can be remembered via the acronym SAMCEL(S):

- **Sleep**
- **Appetite**
- **Memory**
- **Concentration**
- **Energy**
- **Libido**

Plus
- **Suicidal ideations**

Plus ID
- **Interest lost in life activities**
- **Depressed mood**

Utilizing SAMCEL(S) at each individual session helps assess the individual in a rapid, logical, organized fashion providing a clearer global perspective and a record of the individual's progress. SAMCEL(S) plus ID capture the criteria for major depressive disorder found in the *Diagnostic and Statistical Manual of Mental Disorders, 4th Edition-TR*.

In typical depression, the individual will describe difficulty falling asleep, loss of appetite, decrease in memory and concentration, energy that is nervous and nonproductive, and loss of libido. Suicidal thoughts may or may not be present. In atypical depression, individuals describe excessive sleepiness, excessive appetite, decrease in memory and concentration, absence of energy, and loss of libido. Suicidal thoughts may or may not be present (Table 1). The 3 important distinguishing elements of atypical depression are:

- Hypersomnia (excessive sleeping)
- Hyperphagia (excessive eating)
- Anergia (lack of energy)

Table 1. Typical Versus Atypical Depression: Assessing the 6 Neurovegetative Functioning Inventory Indices

Indices	Typical Depression	Atypical Depression
Sleep	⇓ Individual reports thinking all night about what is bothering him or her	⇑⇑ Individual reports sleeping all the time and awakening still tired
Appetite	⇓	⇑⇑ Individual reports being on the "see-food diet": I see food and I eat it
Memory	⇓	⇓
Concentration	⇓	⇓
Energy	⇑ Individual reports increased nonproductive energy	⇓⇓ Individual describes feeling like a slug
Libido	⇓	⇓
Suicidal ideations	+/0 Individual may or may not have suicidal thoughts	+/0 Individual may or may not have suicidal thoughts

⇑= increase; ⇑⇑ = dramatic increase; ⇓ = decrease; and ⇓⇓ = dramatic decrease.

Treating Depression with Medication

Note: Before initiating any therapy, the clinician should obtain informed consent from the patient, parent, or guardian (see Appendix 1).

To understand the use of antidepressant medications, it is important to understand the biological theory of depression, in particular, the monoamine hypothesis. This theory proposes that depression results from a deficiency in 1 or more of 3 neurotransmitters, dopamine, norepinephrine, and/or serotonin.

Neurotransmitters are naturally occurring chemicals found in the neurons in the brain. These chemicals allow electrical impulses to be communicated from one neuron to the next via chemical conversion and transfer. The neuron before the synapse releases a chemical into the synapse to continue the signal to the postsynaptic neuron where it is reconverted to an electrical impulse (Figure 2). This is the process that mediates thought, mood, and motor activity.

In summary:
- Neurons serve as the electrical highway for the communication of mood, thought, and movement.
- Between neurons there is a space called the synaptic cleft, or synapse. On each side of this space is a neuron. The neuron before the synapse is the presynaptic neuron; on the other side of the synapse is the postsynaptic neuron.
- Within the presynaptic neuron are:
  - The reuptake pump
  - Monoamine oxidase disassemblers that destroy the neurotransmitter returned to the neuron by the reuptake pump
  - A neurotransmitter production factory that combines substrates to build the neurotransmitters to be placed into vesicles
  - Vesicles, where the neurotransmitters waiting to be released into the synapse are stored
  - The neurotransmitter that is released into the synapse to find its way to the awaiting postsynaptic receptor sites
- The neurotransmitter released by the presynaptic neuron binds into the postsynaptic receptor sites found on the postsynaptic neuron.

Depletion of specific neurotransmitters results in major depressive disorder, according to the monoamine hypothesis. This depressive state occurs when the presynaptic neuron fails to release the appropriate amount of neurotransmitter into the synapse. One possible cause is overzealous monoamine oxidase disassemblers destroying the neurotransmitter that is brought back into the presynaptic neuron by the reuptake pump. The theory proposes that the postsynaptic neuron up-regulates its receptor sites in order to bind more neurotransmitter because of a depleted amount of presynaptic neurotransmitter.

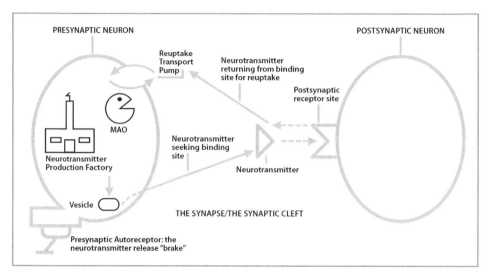

Figure 2. The Monoamine Hypothesis for Major Depressive Disorder.
Neurotransmitter in the presynaptic neuron is released by the vesicle into the synapse. The neurotransmitter moves from the presynaptic neuron through the synapse toward the postsynaptic receptor site where it binds. On binding, the message that it carries is delivered. That message is reconverted from a chemical signal back into an electrical signal. The neurotransmitter then disengages from the postsynaptic receptor site to return to the presynaptic neuron. The reuptake transport pump of the presynaptic neuron causes the neurotransmitter to reenter the presynaptic neuron. Once the neurotransmitter reenters the presynaptic neuron, it is at risk of being disassembled by monoamine oxidase (MAO). By releasing the presynaptic autoreceptor brake, inhibiting the reuptake transport pump, and/or inhibiting MAO, more of the neurotransmitter remains available to find an appropriate postsynaptic receptor site to which to bind.

The Cascade Effect of Antidepressant Medication. Because of the cascading process, the antidepressant effect from medication occurs in stages, typically taking from 2 to 6 weeks for improvements in mood to be realized.

When there is dysregulation of the neurotransmission system, mood dysregulation follows. For some reason (hypotheses to follow) the presynaptic neuron is releasing less neurotransmitter into the synapse. As less neurotransmitter is available for the postsynaptic receptor sites on the postsynaptic neuron, the neuron up regulates the number of sites in a vain attempt to capture more neurotransmitter to "normalize" the postsynaptic receptor's function. The up regulation of postsynaptic receptor sites coincides with the ensuing decrease in mood as the postsynaptic receptor fails to receive its needed neurotransmitter supply. The use of an antidepressant medication serves to enhance the supply of neurotransmitter to the postsynaptic neuron by the following steps:

1. The antidepressant medication blocks the presynaptic reuptake transport pump allowing for more neurotransmitter to remain in the synapse and nestle into the postsynaptic receptor sites.
2. Initially this increase in synaptic neurotransmitter reaches the presynaptic neuron's autoreceptor causing this "sensor" to decrease the already minimized presynaptic neuron's release of neurotransmitter.
3. Eventually the presynaptic neuron's autoreceptor is "desensitized" and shuts down, allowing for the free release of neurotransmitter into the synapse.
4. As this "flood" of neurotransmitter occurs into the synapse, the postsynaptic receptor sites become inundated with neurotransmitter, leading to their down regulation as the postsynaptic neuron becomes properly re-nourished and mood returns to "normal."
   - Neurotransmitter dysfunction-→Up regulation Postsynaptic Receptor Sites→ Mood Decline
   - Antidepressant Medication→Blockade of Presynaptic Reuptake Transport Pump→Neurotransmitter release initiates presynaptic autoreceptor "brake" on presynaptic neurotransmitter release
   - Desensitization of autoreceptor→free release of neurotransmitter→ flooding postsynaptic receptor sites
   - Postsynaptic neuron "normalizes"→Postsynaptic receptor sites down regulate→Mood stabilizes/Depression Improves

The 3 Key Neurotransmitters in Treating Depression. The 3 main neurotransmitter systems in the central nervous system responsible for neurotransmitter-mediated depression and/or its treatment are dopamine, norepinephrine (noradrenaline), and serotonin (5-hydroxytryptamine, or 5HT).

Dopamine is found in 4 major brain pathways. The mesolimbic pathway impacts mood and pleasure; the mesocortical pathway impacts motivation and emotional response; the nigrostriatal pathway impacts smooth motor function; and the tuberoinfundibular pathway impacts prolactin levels. The production of dopamine begins with the amino acid tyrosine. Tyrosine hydroxylase converts tyrosine into dihydroxy-phenyl-alanine (DOPA). This is converted by DOPA decarboxylase into dopamine.

$$\text{Tyrosine} \xrightarrow{\text{Tyrosine hydroxylase}} \text{DOPA} \xrightarrow{\text{DOPA decarboxylase}} \text{Dopamine}$$

Currently, 5 main dopamine receptors have been identified: D_1, D_2, D_3, D_4, and D_5. The most investigated of these are the D_2 and D_4 receptor sites. The D_2 receptor site is stimulated by dopaminergic agonists for the treatment of

Parkinson's disease and blocked by dopamine antagonist medications (antipsychotic medications) for the treatment of psychosis/schizophrenia.

Norepinephrine is produced in the noradrenergic neurons. As with dopamine, tyrosine is the amino acid precursor for norepinephrine. It is transported into the central nervous system from the blood by means of an active transport pump. Once tyrosine is moved into the neuron, 3 enzymes act on it. Tyrosine hydroxylase serves as the rate-limiting and most important enzyme in the regulation of norepinephrine synthesis. It is this enzyme that converts the amino acid tyrosine into DOPA. Then DOPA decarboxylase converts DOPA into dopamine. Finally, dopamine beta hydroxylase converts dopamine into norepinephrine.

$$\text{Tyrosine} \xrightarrow{\text{Tyrosine hydroxylase}} \text{DOPA} \xrightarrow{\text{DOPA decarboxylase}} \text{Dopamine}$$

$$\text{Dopamine} \xrightarrow{\text{Dopamine beta hydroxylase}} \text{Norepinephrine}$$

Norepinephrine is stored in vesicles in the presynaptic neuron. A nerve impulse sends it from the presynaptic neuron into the synapse and on to an awaiting postsynaptic receptor site. Two enzymes destroy norepinephrine, monoamine oxidase (MAO) and catechol O-methyltransferase (COMT).

Serotonin (5HT) is produced from tryptophan in a process that begins when tryptophan is converted into 5-hydroxytryptophan (5HTP) by the enzyme tryptophan hydroxylase. 5HTP is converted into 5HT by the enzyme aromatic amino acid decarboxylase. 5HT is stored in vesicles in the presynaptic neuron until it is released secondary to a neuronal impulse. MAO is the enzyme that destroys/deactivates serotonin.

$$\text{Tryptophan} \xrightarrow{\text{Tryptophan hydroxylase}} \text{5HTP}$$

$$\text{5HTP} \xrightarrow{\text{Aromatic amino acid decarboxylase}} \text{5HT}$$

Numerous 5HT receptor sites exist, with the $5HT_{1A}$ being a presynaptic autoreceptor site that is located on both the cell body and the dendrites. When the $5HT_{1A}$ receptor site, known as the somatodendritic autoreceptor, detects synaptic 5HT, it shuts down the 5HT neuronal impulse flow.

Stimulation of specific 5HT receptor sites is responsible for various common symptoms. For the $5HT_2$ site, these include:

- Agitation
- Akathisia
- Anxiety
- Insomnia
- Panic attacks
- Sexual dysfunction

When the $5HT_3$ site is stimulated, symptoms may include:

- Diarrhea
- Gastrointestinal (GI) distress
- Headache
- Nausea

Norepinephrine can either stimulate serotonin release into the synapse by binding at the postsynaptic $alpha_1$ receptor site or inhibit the release of 5HT by binding at the presynaptic $alpha_2$ receptor site on the 5HT neuron.

A Closer Look at the Classical Antidepressant Medications. Developed in the 1950s, tricyclic antidepressants (TCAs) dominated the treatment scene for depression until 1988 when the serotonin selective reuptake inhibitors (SSRIs) came into the picture.

TCAs effect their result by reuptake pump inhibition. The neurotransmitters are thus able to become more plentiful in the synapse, flooding the awaiting postsynaptic receptor sites. This results in the down-regulation of the up-regulated postsynaptic receptor sites and the resolution of the depressive episode.

TCAs work in a multifaceted way involving the primary inhibition of norepinephrine reuptake and secondary inhibition of 5HT reuptake. Also occurring are anticholinergic, antimuscarinic, and antihistaminergic actions. The TCAs also provide secondary $alpha_1$ adrenergic antagonism. One TCA, Anafranil (clomipramine), demonstrates primary blockade of the reuptake of 5HT along with norepinephrine reuptake blockade.

TCA side effects result from the specific actions of the medications (Box 2). Alpha$_1$ adrenergic blockade can result in

- Decreased blood pressure
- Dizziness
- Drowsiness

Cholinergic blockade (muscarinic) can cause

- Blurry vision
- Confusion/delirium (in the elderly)
- Constipation
- Drowsiness
- Dry mouth
- Urinary retention

Histaminergic blockade commonly brings about

- Drowsiness
- Weight gain

Box 2. Wisdom and Caution in Prescribing Medication(s)

The medications currently available in psychiatry are potent and they can cause side effects. Most have mechanisms of action only partially understood. It is important to proceed cautiously, judiciously, and with clear direction. Some individuals are sensitive responders, who will receive benefit at low doses. Others are rapid responders with rapid onset of benefit. Starting at the lowest dose will allow the medication to clear from the system faster, should the individual experience an allergic response or adverse effect. By starting at the lowest dose and then gently titrating upward, the clinician may be able to avoid side effects altogether as receptor sites and other pathways are slowly and comfortably acclimated to the medication. For individuals who are sensitive responders, starting at the lowest dose and carefully titrating upward allows good response at a dose lower than might be typically used for other individuals.

The TCAs are:

Anafranil (clomipramine)	Pamelor (nortriptyline)
Ascendin (amoxapine)	Sinequan (doxepin)
Elavil (amitriptyline)	Surmontil (trimipramine)
Ludiomil (maprotiline)	Tofranil (imipramine)
Norpramin (desipramine)	Vivactil (protriptyline)

By inhibiting the action of MAO, the MAO inhibitors allow monoamine neurotransmitters to accumulate within the presynaptic neuron. This reverses the deficiency and allows for a more plentiful release of the neurotransmitters, flooding the up-regulated postsynaptic receptor sites and causing them to down-regulate. Consistent with the monoamine theory, as the up-regulated postsynaptic receptor sites down-regulate, the depression subsides.

Tyramine is an amine that is present in food, especially wine and aged cheeses, and acts to increase the release of norepinephrine. Under normal circumstances, MAO gobbles up the excess norepinephrine released by tyramine. However, if an MAO inhibitor is given to an individual and the individual is also consuming foods high in tyramine, excess norepinephrine may be released, leading to dangerous elevations of blood pressure.

The most common side effects caused by the MAO inhibitors are:

• Dietary interactions
• Medication interactions
• Insomnia
• Orthostatic hypotension
• Sexual dysfunction
• Weight gain

The traditional oral MAO inhibitors are Marplan (isocarboxazid), Nardil (phenelzine), and Parnate (tranylcypromine).

In 2006, the US Food and Drug Administration (FDA) approved Emsam (selegiline), an MAO inhibitor delivered through the skin via a transdermal patch that is changed daily. This medication, available as a 6-mg, 9-mg, and 12-mg patch, is absorbed over a 24-hour period. With the active ingredient being absorbed through the skin instead of by oral ingestion, the first-pass effect is avoided. The first-pass effect refers to oral medications that enter the digestive tract and are carried through portal circulation to the liver. In the liver the medication is metabolized and, depending on the medication involved, a decreased amount of the original compound is then available. Medications introduced directly into the blood circulation either by injection or transdermal patch avoid this hepatic metabolism.

A Closer Look at the SSRIs. The SSRIs begin their cascade of benefit at the $5HT_{1a}$ somatodendritic presynaptic receptor site. At this autoreceptor, down-regulation takes place and the axon terminal releases large amounts of 5HT. The 5HT traverses the synapse to attach to the postsynaptic receptor sites. The presynaptic reuptake transport pump is also blocked, maintaining more 5HT in the synapse. As the postsynaptic neuron normalizes with the new influx of vital neurotransmitter, the up regulated postsynaptic receptor sites down regulate heralding the stabilization and "normalization" of mood. The bioactivity of SSRIs can lead to various side affects. For example, there is the potential for SSRI-induced akathisia. 5HT inhibits dopamine release in the basal ganglia, so when prescribing SSRIs, clinicians should monitor for possible extra-pyramidal effects.

The SSRIs also have the potential to create insomnia. Stimulating $5HT_2$ disrupts slow wave sleep. This can induce nocturnal myoclonus, which can increase the frequency of nocturnal awakenings.

5HT tends to inhibit sexual functioning, while dopamine tends to enhance it. 5HT antagonizes dopamine, and blocking dopamine leads to increased levels of prolactin. The medications that enhance dopamine, in particular Wellbutrin (bupropion), often reverse SSRI-induced sexual dysfunction. Clinical evidence supports the hypothesis that the $5HT_2$ pathway is the cause of sexual dysfunction secondary to the use of SSRIs. $5HT_2$-antagonizing antidepressants do not cause sexual dysfunction. Remeron (mirtazapine) blocks both the $5HT_2$ and $5HT_3$ pathways, so clinicians may prescribe it along with an SSRI. It is the blockade of $5HT_2$ that allows the addition of mirtazapine to offset the sexual side effects, as well as offsetting insomnia and jitteriness.

When $5HT_3$ receptors, which are located in the wall of the gut, are stimulated, they increase GI motility. Initially, SSRIs may cause GI cramps and diarrhea. Mirtazapine, which blocks both the $5HT_2$ and $5HT_3$ pathways, can be prescribed as an adjunct to an SSRI to offset the initial GI side effects, as well as headaches caused by activation of the $5HT_3$ pathway. The receptors are desensitized to the side effects typically within 2 weeks, at which time mirtazapine can be discontinued.

Available SSRIs. The SSRI revolution began in 1983 in Europe, with the introduction of Luvox (fluvoxamine), followed in 1986 by Celexa (citalopram). In the United States, Eli Lilly began marketing Prozac (fluoxetine) in 1988. As of 2009, the SSRI choices are Celexa (citalopram), Luvox (fluvoxamine), Paxil (paroxetine), Prozac (fluoxetine), Zoloft (sertraline), and Lexapro (escitalopram), which is the only SSRI without a generic version.

- **Celexa (citalopram)** is the progenitor of escitalopram, and like escitalopram, it has a high affinity for the 5HT reuptake pump and low potential for side effects. Citalopram is user-friendly with regard to the cytochrome P_{450} enzymatic clearinghouse of the liver and has minimal potential for discontinuation syndrome. The most frequent side effect of citalopram clinically reported is increased perspiring on exertion. It has a low potential to cause sexual dysfunction or weight gain.

- **Lexapro (escitalopram)** is the S-enantiomer of the citalopram molecule. It is the "cleaner, leaner citalopram." It demonstrates a more rapid onset of benefit, within 1 to 2 weeks. Escitalopram is typically initiated as 10 mg, thought to be equivalent to 20 to 40 mg of citalopram. Escitalopram is also available in a 5-mg pill, which may be taken for several days with upward titration to 10 mg as tolerated. For elderly individuals or individuals presenting specifically with generalized anxiety disorder, escitalopram can be started at 2.5 mg with upward titration as clinically indicated. As of March 2009, its use for treating adolescents aged 12 to 17 years for major depressive disorder was FDA approved.

- **Luvox (fluvoxamine)** is used for depression in Europe. In the United States it has only been approved specifically for obsessive-compulsive disorder. As it has the potential to be sedating, it is best taken at night. The 2 SSRIs with the least potential for sexual dysfunction are the 2 Ls: Lexapro and Luvox. In March 2008, the FDA approved the long-acting formulation of Luvox as Luvox CR for the treatment of social anxiety disorder and obsessive-compulsive disorder. In an agreement between Solvay Pharmaceuticals and Jazz Pharmaceuticals, Jazz is marketing Luvox CR.

- **Paxil (paroxetine)/Paxil CR** is thought to have a bit more sedation potential than the other SSRIs and has potential to cause weight gain. Paroxetine provides rapid benefit for calming anxiety. The controlled-release version has fewer side effects, including less potential for weight gain, than its immediate-release progenitor.

- **Prozac (fluoxetine)** is FDA approved in children and adolescents (ages 7 to 17 years) for major depressive disorder and OCD. Typically, out of 10 people, 7 to 8 will find it activating, 1 will find it sedating and 1 will see no difference. While at initiation it does not facilitate sleep, after about 2 weeks, it should begin to normalize the individual's sleep patterns. Prozac's activating quality does not calm nervousness initially; however, it calms anxiety after about 2 weeks.

- **Zoloft (sertraline)** is FDA approved for treating major depressive disorder, obsessive-compulsive disorder, panic disorder, post-traumatic stress disorder, and premenstrual dysphoric disorder. Out of every 10 individuals for whom it is prescribed, 4 will find sertraline activating, 4 will find it mildly to moderately sedating, and 2 will see no difference. As a result, it may facilitate sleep and/or provide daytime agitated energy improvement.

While the SSRIs are thought to be safer and better tolerated than the older line MAO inhibitors and TCAs, in clinical trials the newer medications have not been shown to surpass the classical antidepressants in effectiveness. The edge these newer medications possess is their safer side effect profiles. Because of safer, milder, and fewer side effects, individual compliance is better and thus there is a greater likelihood of achieving remission of depression, compared with older medications. Put simply, when individuals take their medication, they have a greater chance of getting better.

The Next Generation of Antidepressants. A number of other antidepressants are available to treat depression.

- **Cymbalta (duloxetine)**, developed as a dual action medication in the vein of Effexor XR (venlafaxine), differs from venlafaxine in that it blocks the presynaptic reuptake transport pumps of 5HT and norepinephrine equally. This medication is a 50/50 reuptake transport pump inhibitor of both neurotransmitters. As the dose is increased, the blockade of both neurotransmitter reuptake pumps increases equally. The dosing range is from 20 to 60 mg per day. For women, this medication has very low potential for sexual side effects.

- **Desyrel (trazodone)**, an older line medication, is a $5HT_2$ antagonist as well as a serotonin reuptake inhibitor. Trazodone does not have norepinephrine reuptake inhibition. It has antihistaminergic as well as $alpha_1$ antagonistic properties. Trazodone has long been used as a sleep-inducing medication and is not often used as a first-line antidepressant. It has as a potential side effect, priapism.

- **Effexor XR (venlafaxine)** has trivalent benefit potential. At its lower range (37.5 to 75 mg), it is an SSRI, blocking the presynaptic reuptake transport pump for 5HT. As the dose is increased to the range of 112.5 to 150 mg, the serotonergic benefit is joined by the presynaptic reuptake transport pump inhibition of norepinephrine. Beyond 225 mg, inhibition of the reuptake transport pump for dopamine also occurs (Table 2). At the higher ranges of dosing, venlafaxine has the potential to raise blood pressure. Instead of taking venlafaxine up to its higher range, the individual can take it to its dosage midrange (from 112.5 to 150 mg) and then add Wellbutrin XL (bupropion). With the addition of bupropion, the individual receives the dopaminergic benefit without the weight gain or blood pressure elevation potential of venlafaxine. The addition of bupropion often offsets the SSRI-induced sexual dysfunction.

Table 2. Actions of Venlafaxine

Dose	37.5–75 mg	112.5–187.5 mg	225–300 mg
Medication type action	SSRI	SSRI + TCA	SSRI + TCA + bupropion
Reuptake transport pump inhibition	Serotonin	Serotonin + norepinephrine	Serotonin + norepinephrine + dopamine

Abbreviations: SSRI, serotonin selective reuptake inhibitor; TCA, tricyclic antidepressant.

- **Nefazodone**, a cousin to trazodone, FDA approved in December of 1994, is a serotonin antagonist and a reuptake inhibitor. It acts by potent blockade of $5HT_2$ receptors, inhibition of 5HT reuptake, and inhibition of norepinephrine reuptake. This medication works presynaptically at the reuptake pump as well as postsynaptically at the $5HT_2$ receptor site. Nefazodone has been found to be beneficial in depression that has comorbid anxiety, agitation, and insomnia, or prior SSRI-induced sexual dysfunction.

A potential risk with use of nefazodone is the mCPP metabolite. Four percent of the Caucasian population lacks the cytochrome P_{450} enzyme of 2D6. Because of this lack of 2D6, treatment with an SSRI will result in the formation of the metabolite mCPP. This leads to stimulation rather than blockade of the $5HT_{2A}/5HT_{2C}$ receptors. If nefazodone is then prescribed, the effect is the opposite of its desired result and may include agitation, dizziness and/or lightheadedness, insomnia, and nausea.

These effects can usually be avoided by providing a wash-out period whenever it is necessary to change therapy between an SSRI and nefazodone. The recommended procedure is to discontinue the first medication (either an SSRI or nefazodone) and wait 2 full weeks before initiating the new therapy (nefazodone or an SSRI).

Another risk is the LSD-like side effect, palinopsia. Palinopsia is a visual phenomenon, referred to as visual trailing, in which there is continued visual perception of an object after the actual stimulus of the object has left the eyes' visual field. Bristol Myers Squibb discontinued marketing Serzone in the US and Canada on May 20th, 2004 due to reports of acute hepatotoxicity. The medication is currently available only as the generic nefazodone, and has continued use for individuals for whom it was the only medication to provide benefit.

- **Pristiq (desvenlafaxine)** was approved on February 29, 2008 for the treatment of major depressive disorder, social anxiety disorder and panic disorder. It is a once a day long acting antidepressant dosed at 50mg. While it was introduced with 50mg as the starting dose and treatment dose, clinicians have been increasing the dose to 100mg and 150mg as necessary in treating individuals with depressive disorder.

- **Remeron (mirtazapine)** works to enhance serotonergic activity without the side effects often encountered with the classical SSRIs. Mirtazapine is an antidepressant medication with multiple mechanisms of action. First, it is an alpha$_2$ antagonist. By blocking the presynaptic alpha$_2$ receptor site, norepinephrine does not inhibit its own release. Thus, more norepinephrine is released and the blockade of the postsynaptic alpha$_2$ receptor sites causes the release of serotonin. Second, mirtazapine blocks the 5HT$_2$ and 5HT$_3$ receptors. The blockade of these 2 serotonin receptors counteracts the potential for the serotonergic side effects of GI upset, jitteriness, headache, and sexual dysfunction. Finally, mirtazapine is a histamine$_1$ antagonist. The histamine$_1$ blockade counteracts the anxiogenic effects of norepinephrine release, while giving mirtazapine its sedating, appetite enhancing, and weight increasing side effect.

The sedation, appetite enhancement, and weight gain occur at lower doses. In the right individual this can be beneficial when inability to sleep and/or recent weight loss is an issue. The sedation and weight gain are thought to be inversely related to the dose: the lower the dose, the more sedating/weight inducing; the higher the dose, the less sedating and weight inducing. Therefore, if the medication proves too sedating or stimulates too much weight gain at 15 mg, increasing the dose to 30 or 45 mg can reduce these actions. As noted above, mirtazapine may also serve as an adjunctive medication to control SSRI side effects, including insomnia, GI upset/nausea, and sexual dysfunction.

• **Wellbutrin IR/SR/XL (bupropion)** is a non-SSRI that is also marketed under the brand name Zyban. It blocks the reuptake transport pump for dopamine and has mild reuptake pump inhibition of norepinephrine, making it dual action. Improving focus and concentration, as well as energy, bupropion is also used adjunctively with SSRIs to offset sexual dysfunction and reverse SSRI poop-out. Bupropion serves as a stand-alone antidepressant when dopamine is the key neurotransmitter in resolving the individual's depression. It is thought to be the magic bullet for atypical depression because the medication offsets increased sleeping (offsets hypersomnia), calms over-eating(offsets hyperphagia), improves energy (offsets anergia), and improves focus and concentration. Wellbutrin is available in immediate release (IR), sustained release (SR), and extended release (XL) formulations. This medication is used both as a stand-alone antidepressant and as an adjunctive medication in combination with the SSRIs and venlafaxine.

• **An Off-Label Adjunct – Provigil (modafinil)** is an energy-enhancing medication that is currently FDA approved for excessive daytime sleepiness associated with narcolepsy, obstructive sleep apnea/hypopnea syndrome, and shift-work sleep disorder. It is currently used off-label to offset the residual sleepiness and fatigue that often occur in depressed individuals and for the medication-induced fatigue of individuals taking antipsychotic medications. It is used adjunctively off-label to enhance the mood benefits of antidepressant medications. It has benefit for reestablishing energy and improving focus and concentration. For individuals with a milder variant of depression not meeting the criteria for major depressive disorder, modafinil is being used off-label to treat what is being called mild or minor depression.

Focus the Medication Selection. SAMCEL(S) can help focus the selection of a medication to treat depression. Assessing the 6 neurovegetative functioning inventory indices gives the clinician an indication as to which direction to follow:

- Is sleep too little or too much? Evaluate a medication for its energizing or sedating effects (Box 3).
- Is appetite too little or too much? Consider medications based on their ability to stimulate or to help curb appetite.
- Is memory or concentration compromised? Choose from among the medications thought to improve memory/concentration.
- Is energy decreased or increased? Again, attention should be given toward selecting a medication based on its energizing or sedating effects.
- Is libido decreased or increased? Some medications may have libido-enhancing effects, while others may help to calm the libidinous impulse or slow the response from arousal to climax.

Box 3. Making the Most of Side Effects

In his third law of motion, Sir Isaac Newton proposed that "for every action there is an equal and opposite reaction." To paraphrase Sir Isaac Newton and to apply his concept to medication, "For every benefit of a medication there is the potential for equal and opposite risks and side effects."

Side effects are the bane of medicine. Once a side effect is experienced, individuals are less willing to continue on the medication or try another one. When possible, the prescribing clinician should use potential side effect(s) as a benefit. If the individual is not sleeping, look for an antidepressant medication that has the side effect of sedation. If the individual is not eating, look for an antidepressant medication that will increase appetite. For individuals who have lost all energy, look for an antidepressant medication that has the side effect of being energizing.

Consider Comorbidities. Mood disorders are not always discrete in their occurrence, as they may appear with other psychiatric or medical conditions. After the clinician assesses the neurovegetative functioning inventory indices, it is important to ask additional questions to identify potential comorbid conditions that may affect the choice of medication and the dose at which it is given. These supplemental questions include:

- Is the individual anxious?
- Does the individual have comorbid conditions such as
  - Attention-deficit hyperactivity disorder
  - Eating disorders
  - Enuresis
  - Nicotine dependence
  - Obsessive-compulsive disorder
  - Seizure disorder
  - Sleep disorders
  - Substance abuse/dependence
  - Thought disorder
  - Tic disorders
  - Weight issues (overweight or underweight)

Bipolar disorder is discussed in greater detail later in this chapter. When assessing an individual for major depressive disorder, the clinician should determine whether the individual's presentation with depressive symptoms is indicative of a unipolar depression or reflects an underlying bipolar disorder for which the hypomanic or manic episodes have remained unobserved. The 3 main types of bipolar disorder may all include depressive episodes, with type I being defined as manic episodes with or without depressive episodes; type II as at least 1 hypomanic episode with depressive episodes; and type III (mixed) experiencing agitation, depression, and mania.

For individuals experiencing a depressive episode, antidepressant medications can have 2 potential adverse impacts. First, a manic-like episode may occur by mere happenstance when the individual takes the medication. This is termed an *iatrogenic occurrence*, meaning it is medication induced. Second, the medication may unmask an underlying bipolar disorder that has previously neither declared itself nor been diagnosed.

Evaluate Physical, Social, and Medical Factors When Prescribing Medications. Because of the profound effects antidepressant (and other) medications can have on an individual physically and emotionally, the clinician needs to take a wide range of factors into consideration before prescribing (Box 4). Chapter 12 outlines the interview process in greater detail. Key factors to evaluate before writing a prescription are:

- Age of the individual: Metabolic rates vary by age. Consider body mass based on age also.
- Allergies/comorbid medical conditions
- Belief/placebo effect
- Cost issues for the individual, which can impact compliance
- Employment/school as it applies to drug testing (amphetamines) and daily dosing regimen. Elementary or high school students may bristle at multiple daily dosing during the school day because of embarrassment over having to report to the office or school nurse for medication. Sustained release/extended release forms of the medication(s), if available, may be preferable to avoid having to take medication at school.
- Enhancing serotonin may decrease or block dopamine, leading to SSRI-induced extrapyramidal side effects.
- Family history/previous response to medication
- FDA approved approaches versus off-label uses
- SSRI poop-out. For an unknown reason the medication may lose effectiveness. This typically occurs about 2 years into the medication regimen.

Box 4. Goldman's Law of Medicine

When it comes to initiating a medication approach, it is still trial and error within educated parameters. *Goldman's Law of Medicine:*

THE FOUNDATION OF MEDICINE IS SCIENCE – THE APPLICATION OF THAT SCIENCE IS ART

BIPOLAR DISORDER: CLINICAL TIPS AND PEARLS FOR DIAGNOSIS AND TREATMENT

According to the National Institute of Mental Health, 2.2 million American adults suffer from bipolar disorder. While the onset of bipolar disorder typically occurs in late adolescence or the early 20s, it can occur in the third decade as well as in childhood.

The 3 types of bipolar disorder are:

- Type I – Mania with or without a major depressive episode
- Type II –At least one major depressive episode with at least 1 episode of hypomania
- Mixed –Symptoms of depressed mood and agitation/mania concurrently

Diagnosing Bipolar Disorder

The key to treating bipolar disorder is diagnosing it. While this may seem obvious, the condition is often treated as depression, anxiety, or irritability and impulsivity before being clearly diagnosed as bipolar disorder. In youngsters, the child/adolescent may be diagnosed and treated first for attention-deficit/hyperactivity disorder before bipolar disorder is either suspected or clearly defined. Some clinicians postulate that attention-deficit/hyperactivity disorder may be a premorbid condition evolving into bipolar disorder.

Making the diagnosis of bipolar disorder is not easy. There are many confounders. In an outpatient practice, individuals typically do not present in either the hypomanic or full-blown manic stages. First, hypomania is pleasurable and productive. Individuals are getting too much work done and are feeling too good about it to take the time to come to the clinician's office. They also don't feel anything is wrong when they are hypomanic. By the time they are fully manic, they are not going to come in to an outpatient practice. Instead, they are typically transported by family or police to the nearest emergency department for evaluation and hospitalization because they are out of control (Box 5). Thus, individuals typically come into the clinician's office when they are depressed. When the clinician only sees the individual in depressed stages, it is difficult to discern bipolar disorder. This in fact is the reason so many bipolar individuals are diagnosed with and treated for unipolar depression. Unfortunately, individuals with bipolar disorder type I are at risk of being pushed into mania when they are prescribed an antidepressant medication. Furthermore, a depressed individual with bipolar disorder type II is unlikely to receive full benefit when treated with an antidepressant.

Making an accurate diagnosis requires:

1. *A thorough family history.* Bipolar disorder typically does not occur de novo. There is usually a strong generational family history of this disease.
2. *A thorough past psychiatric history of the individual.* This includes past hospitalizations, past and current medications, and history of response to the

Box 5. Individual Safety

Severe depressive episodes with psychotic features and full-blown manic episodes result in distortions of thought processes and disruptions of judgment. These distortions can lead to irrational behaviors compromising the individual's safety and the safety of those around him or her. The bipolar individual suffering from a severe depressive episode may entertain suicidal ideations; 1 in 2 individuals with bipolar disorder will attempt suicide at least once in their lifetime and 1 in 5 will succeed. Full-blown manic episodes can lead to paranoid ideations that result in behaviors that may put others at risk. Full-blown mania with racing thoughts can result in impulsive behaviors that prove dangerous to both the individual and others. These distortions of thought and resulting disruptions of behavior may necessitate immediate hospitalization for safety and stabilization. Some individuals become so disorganized that they are unable to care for their daily needs. If safety is an issue, then hospitalization is warranted.

medications. Bipolar individuals typically have had multiple past hospitalizations and have a "laundry list" of medications that were tried, with varied effectiveness, before a successful combination was found. They are likely to have been prescribed several current medications, which they stopped taking, leading to their current bipolar episode.

3. *A thorough social history.* Bipolar individuals often have a history of multiple jobs and marriages. There may be past legal issues such as traffic violations, driving while intoxicated, or disorderly conduct arrests.

The clinician should assess SAMCEL(S), the 6 neurovegetative functioning inventory indices plus ask about suicidal/homicidal thoughts, to assist in the diagnosis:

- Sleep in individuals with bipolar disorder may be disturbed at each of the poles, both at the highs of mania and the lows of depression. Individuals experiencing either hypomania or full-blown mania will find they do not need the usual and customary amount of sleep. They will be able to go without sleep for 1 or several nights and still be fully charged during the day. When the mood declines into depression, on the other hand, sleep swings to the other extreme, with individuals finding they may be sleeping excessively, as the bed becomes a hiding place from daily activities.

- Appetite may be either increased or decreased in any of the mood fluctuations. Individuals who are depressed may become hyperphagic, using food as a means to comfort the decreased mood, or they may feel too distressed to eat at all. When moods are elevated, these individuals may consume more food as they celebrate life excessively, or they may not eat, being too energized and active to even think of eating.

- Memory and concentration are disrupted in depressed moods. While memory and concentration may seem improved to the hypomanic and manic individual, in reality, memory and concentration may show signs of decline to an independent observer. The racing thoughts of mania disrupt orderly thinking and concentration.

- Energy is either nervous and nonproductive in the typically depressed individual or completely depleted in the atypically depressed individual, resulting in anergia. In the hypomanic individual, energy begins to increase; in the manic individual, energy becomes exaggerated.

- Libido is decreased in individuals with depression and often mildly to wildly elevated as the individual moves from hypomania to full-blown mania. In the adolescent with depression, the libido may be increased.

- Suicidal ideations may or may not be present in either depressed or bipolar individuals. Individuals suffering from depression have a 15% suicide rate, compared to a 20% suicide rate in bipolar individuals.

Determining the Type of Bipolar Disorder. Before selecting a medication to treat the disorder, the clinician must first determine whether the individual is suffering from type I, type II, or mixed bipolar disorder. This is important because the medications used may vary among types. Type I bipolar disorder is hallmarked by the full-blown manic episode. It is imperative not to use an antidepressant without a major mood stabilizer in place. Prescribing an antidepressant medication without a concurrent major mood stabilizing medication creates the risk of causing a manic episode. In type I bipolar disorder, a major mood stabilizer should be prescribed first, thus placing a ceiling on the elevated mood; an antidepressant can then be added to elevate the lowered mood floor, the depression.

Type II bipolar disorder is hallmarked by several depressive episodes with at least 1 hypomanic episode. As noted above, the clinician is unlikely to see the individual in the hypomanic state. The individual will present when depressed. Depression is painful, while hypomania is not. For the type II bipolar individual, prescribing a major mood stabilizer will preclude hypomanic episodes; then to avoid depressive episodes, an antidepressant medication can be added. In order to establish bipolar type II as a diagnosis, it is important to ask the following questions:

- Do you ever experience periods of elevated mood where you feel a little happier than usual with more energy and needing less sleep?
- Do you ever have episodes of being more energetic and mildly irritable at the same time?
- Do you ever have episodes where you have more energy during the day, need less sleep at night, and don't feel tired or fatigued the next day?
- Is there any history in your family of bipolar disorder?
- Do friends or family ever remark that you seem overly happy or too energetic?

The mixed type of bipolar disorder is seen least often. Once seen, it is always remembered. The individual experiences both a manic episode and a major depressive episode at the same time. This individual is sad and crying, laughing and expansive, angry and irritable, all in the same day. To meet the criteria for this diagnosis, these episodes should occur most of the day, every day, for at least 7 days.

Medicating Bipolar Disorder

Preparing for Medication. Having made the diagnosis of bipolar disorder, the clinician next needs to lay the groundwork for initiating psychotropic medication. The initial step is to establish baseline laboratory values. Individual responses to major mood stabilizers vary, so medication approaches may need to be changed until an effective treatment approach is found. Because different medications clear through different organ systems and affect these organ systems differently, obtaining full baseline laboratory values is justified and indicated.

- **Baseline Complete Blood Count**. Obtaining a complete blood count can eliminate as a diagnosis diseases that can mimic bipolar disorder. For example, anemia can mimic the fatigue and malaise of depression, and an infectious disease can disturb cognition and mood. Furthermore, some medications have hematologic effects that need monitoring. Lithium can elevate the white blood cell count, and other major mood stabilizers can adversely impact the bone marrow's ability to produce new blood cells.

- **Baseline Kidney Function**. Obtaining baseline values for blood urea nitrogen (BUN) and creatinine will establish kidney function for future comparisons. Lithium clears through the kidneys and can adversely impact kidney function. When the individual is being treated with lithium BUN and creatinine levels should be checked every 6 months for the first 2 years, then annually thereafter.

- **Baseline Liver Function**. Most of the major mood stabilizers clear through the liver and can adversely impact liver function. It is important to assess baseline liver function, because hepatic encephalopathy can cause disturbances in cognition and can mimic mood and thought disorders.

- **Baseline Pancreas Function (Amylase/Lipase)**. The single presenting symptom of a tumor of the head of the pancreas may be depression, so it is important to rule out pancreatic dysfunction when a mood disorder is being assessed. Furthermore, baseline pancreas laboratory values can be compared with subsequent readings to assess acute pancreatitis, an effect of many of the major mood stabilizers.

- **Baseline Thyroid Function**. Both hypothyroid and hyperthyroid function can mimic many of the symptoms of depression and bipolar disorder; assessing thyroid function by measuring thyroid-stimulating hormone levels enables the clinician to rule out confounding thyroid disease. Lithium can disrupt thyroid function, so thyroid function should be measured every 6 months for 2 years, then annually thereafter, when lithium is prescribed.

Selecting the Medication – The Classical Approach. Lithium is FDA approved for treating acute episodes of bipolar disorder and as prophylaxis for recurrent episodes. Its effectiveness in treating mood instability was first discovered in 1948 by the Australian psychiatrist John F. J. Cade. Since then, it has been considered the gold standard for treating bipolar disorder, although today a myriad of other medications are equally successful as first-line approaches. Individuals taking lithium must be closely monitored for signs of lithium toxicity. The therapeutic range should be 0.5 to1.2 mEq/L. If an individual becomes dehydrated, the lithium can become concentrated and potentially toxic. Diarrhea, vomiting, or excessive perspiring can cause dehydration. In addition, lithium itself is known to cause polydypsia, which is excessive fluid intake, and polyuria, which is excessive urination. Other side effects of taking lithium include weight gain and exacerbation of psoriasis and acne. Taking the long-acting formulations often helps avoid the metallic taste experienced by some individuals, as well as allowing individuals to avoid GI upset. Lithium can cause diabetes insipidus, lead to renal failure, slow thyroid function, cause inversion of T-waves on an ECG, and cause an elevation of the white count as seen on the complete blood count lab.

Selecting the Medication – A Newer Approach, Antiseizure Medications. A number of medications approved to prevent seizures are also approved and effective in treating bipolar disorder:

- **Depakote (divalproex sodium/valproic acid)** requires serum levels to be monitored; its therapeutic range is 50 to 125 µg/mL. Potential side effects include weight gain and skin rash. As the rash indicates a potential for Stevens-Johnson syndrome, which can be fatal, divalproex sodium should be discontinued in the presence of any rash. Also, female individuals may develop polycystic ovary syndrome. The potential for bone marrow suppression requires monitoring the reticulocyte count. For acute mania, the recommended dosing is 10 to 15 mg/kg by mouth per day in divided doses 3 times a day. If the extended release version is prescribed, the dose for acute mania is 25 mg/kg per day for acute stabilization.

- **Keppra (levetiracetam)** is an antiseizure medication that is being used off-label for treating mood lability and bipolar disorder. Levetiracetam can be prescribed in adolescents and adults, although not in children. Some children may become over-activated with this medication instead of being calmed. Initially, the dose is 250 mg by mouth at night for several nights and then it is increased to 250 mg by mouth twice a day for at least a week, at which time the response should be reassessed. Levetiracetam is dosed clinically, not based on serum levels, so there is no need for blood tests.

- **Lamictal (lamotrigine)** is FDA approved for treating bipolar disorder. Studies have shown it to be effective in treating the depressive component of type II bipolar disorder as well. Dosing lamotrigine should start low and be titrated slowly upward. In adolescents and adults, lamotrigine should be started at 25 mg by mouth once a day for 2 weeks, then increased to 25 mg twice a day for 2 weeks. After 2 weeks at 25mg BID, if needed, the medication dose can be increased by 25 mg every 7 to 10 days. Many individuals will see improvement with doses as low as 25 mg twice a day, while others reach benefit at 50 mg twice a day. Many clinicians recommend reaching 100 mg twice a day. The most significant side effect to monitor is a skin rash, which has the potential to become Stevens-Johnson syndrome. If the individual has reached a dose of 25 mg twice a day or higher when the rash appears, assess the rash and taper the medication quickly to discontinuation. Individuals on lower doses who develop a rash should discontinue the medication immediately.

- **Tegretol (carbamazepine)** is an antiseizure medication used for mood stabilization that helps improve decreased mood as well. It is metabolized in the liver; baseline liver function studies are indicated with follow-up liver studies every 6 months for the first 2 years, then annually thereafter. Clinicians should monitor for a red skin rash, known as a lobster rash. Carbamazepine can be mildly sedating and has potential to cause weight gain. The clinician should initiate carbamazepine at 100 to 200 mg twice per day and monitor. After 5 days, serum levels should be evaluated and the dose increased, if indicated, by 200 mg per day. The maintenance dosing range is 800 to 1200 mg per day in divided doses 2 to 4 times a day. Its therapeutic range for bipolar disorder is 4 to 12 µg/mL.

- **Topamax (topiramate)** is an antiseizure medication that is being used as a novel or off-label treatment for mood lability and weight management. It is effective in offsetting appetite and facilitating weight loss, and for most individuals, it will calm irritability. However, in some individuals, there may be a paradoxical response of irritability. While some individuals report cognitive dulling at higher dosing ranges such as 200 mg per day, some individuals have reported cognitive dulling at doses as low as 25 mg per day. Some individuals have reported eye pain with associated acute myopia and secondary angle closure glaucoma. Individuals should be advised to inform their clinician immediately should they experience any visual disturbances when taking topiramate. Topiramate is initiated at 25 mg a day for 1 week, then the dosing is assessed and up-titrated to 25 mg twice a day for a week, at which time the clinicians should assess its effectiveness.

- **Trileptal (oxcarbazepine)** is a novel off-label approach to treat bipolar disorder. As with levetiracetam, lamotrigine, and zonisamide, dosage of oxcarbazepine is not based on laboratory serum levels, rather on clinical assessment of benefit. The medication can impact sodium levels causing hyponatremia, so occasional serum sodium checks are prudent. A recommended dosage strategy is: initiate oxcarbazepine at 150 mg by mouth in the evening for 3 to 4 nights and then increase the dose to 150 mg twice a day for a week. Increase by 150 mg every 5 to 7 days, to clinical effectiveness. This can be achieved by going from 150 mg by mouth twice a day to 150 mg in the morning and 300 mg at night, then adding another 150 mg to the morning dose. Once a dose of 300 mg twice a day is achieved, the clinician should observe for 2 weeks and reassess. While the maximum dose for seizures is 2400 mg per day, effectiveness in bipolar disorder is often achieved at 300 to 600 mg twice a day.

- **Zonegran (zonisamide)** is an antiseizure medication that is being used off-label for mood lability and to facilitate weight loss. It comes in doses of 25, 50, and 100 mg, with a maximum daily dose of 600 mg. For calming mood lability and offsetting appetite increase and weight gain, clinically initiating zonisamide at 25 mg a day for 2 weeks, then increasing to twice a day dosing is effective. Weight control can usually be achieved at 25 mg twice a day.

Antiseizure medications should be tapered to discontinuation and not stopped abruptly, as abrupt discontinuation of an antiseizure medication may result in a withdrawal seizure.

Selecting the Medication – The Newest Approach, Atypical Antipsychotic Medications. The atypical antipsychotic medications—Abilify (aripiprazole), Clozaril (clozapine), Geodon (ziprasidone), Risperdal (risperidone), Seroquel (quetiapine), and Zyprexa (olanzapine)—have all been approved for treating the manic episodes of bipolar disorder. While these medications were initially created to treat psychosis, and specifically schizophrenia, their blockade of dopamine is effective in reorganizing thought processes; their blockade of histamine$_1$ provides sedation; and their blockade of the 5HT$_2$ receptor calms feelings of jitteriness and insomnia. These medications are also used off-label to adjunctively enhance the benefit of antidepressant medications (2 medications are used on label, see page 244). When these medications are prescribed, individuals should be monitored for extrapyramidal side effects and metabolic syndrome. In particular, the clinician should monitor for:
- Acute dystonic reaction
- Akathisia
- Neuroleptic malignant syndrome
- Parkinson-like tremor
- Tardive dyskinesia (see Chapter 3)

While the mechanism is not understood nor the actual prevalence known, concern has arisen recently over the development of metabolic syndrome in individuals taking atypical antipsychotic medications. Originally known as syndrome X and insulin resistance syndrome, metabolic syndrome has 5 classic symptoms, 3 or more of which establish the diagnosis:

- Decreased high-density lipoprotein cholesterol (the "good" cholesterol)
- Elevated blood pressure
- Elevated body weight (typically a central obesity with fat deposits predominantly around the waist)
- Elevated serum glucose (increased fasting blood sugars)
- Elevated triglycerides

Recent FDA recommendations are to periodically assess for disruption in glucose metabolism that is thought to be related to the development of diabetes mellitus. The mechanism of action that results in a higher incidence of diabetes in individuals on atypical antipsychotic medications is not currently understood. It may be a function of the psychotic disorders themselves or may be related to some unknown mechanism in the metabolic pathways related to the medications (Box 6). It is also prudent to monitor blood pressure, weight and waist circumference, and cholesterol and triglyceride levels.

Selecting the Medication – Second-line Approaches, the Benzodiazepine Medications. The benzodiazepines have multiple benefits including, calming anxiety, facilitating sleep, offsetting tremor and akathisia, and stopping seizures. If an individual cannot tolerate the major mood stabilizers, the clinician might prescribe a benzodiazepine as a means of controlling mania, in particular Ativan (lorazepam) and Klonopin (clonazepam). Lorazepam is dosed on a regular schedule of 1 to 2 mg 2 to 3 times a day; clonazepam is dosed at 1 to 2 mg twice a day. As with antiseizure medications, if a benzodiazepine medication is abruptly stopped, there is the potential for a withdrawal seizure, so tapering the dose is essential.

OTHER CYCLIC MOOD DISORDERS
Cyclothymic Disorder (Cyclothymia)
Individuals diagnosed with cyclothymic disorder experience at least 2 years of numerous periods of hypomanic symptoms that do not meet the criteria for a manic episode and numerous periods of depressive symptoms that do not meet the criteria for a major depressive episode.

Box 6. Med-Med Interactions

At one time, the goal in psychiatric medication therapy was to treat an individual with one medication, an approach known as monotherapy. However, as research uncovered the biochemical basis of many mental disorders, treatment has focused on selectively targeting specific receptor sites and pathways. This often results in the use of multiple medications for the same individual. In such instances, it is important to understand how medications interact with each other, for example, in the way they are broken down in the body and excreted. The body's utilization of medication with attendant breakdown and excretion of the medication's ingredients is the mechanism called metabolism. The metabolic breakdown of medications occurs through different systems and in different areas of the body, including the brain, intestine, kidney, liver, and lung. The metabolic breakdown of psychiatric medications is most often centered in the cytochrome P_{450} system clearinghouse of the liver. The isoenzymes of this system catalyze oxidative reactions. Because medications will use similar isoenzymes for their metabolic clearance, medications compete to clear the system. When medications compete for clearance, one or more of them may have to wait its turn to be metabolized and serum levels may climb. Alternately, the cytochrome P_{450} system may be speeded up and medication levels may be decreased more rapidly than would be expected. It is these med-med interactions that can be responsible for side effects.

It is important to understand the pathway through which medications clear the body. Some medications clear through the liver (liver clearance) and some clear through the kidneys (renal clearance). If 2 medications are given simultaneously to an individual and both clear through the liver, this increases the load on the liver. On the other hand, if 1 medication clears through the liver and another clears through the kidneys, then neither organ is burdened with an increased load. Thus, sound medical practice calls for obtaining baseline laboratory values for kidney, liver, and thyroid function, as well as conducting periodic monitoring. Comparing the baseline laboratory value with the laboratory value after the medication is taken provides an alert to any negative effect caused by the medications.

Schizoaffective Disorder

Schizoaffective disorder is the combination of thought disturbance and mood disturbance; non-technically it is the comorbidity of bipolar disorder or major depressive disorder and schizophrenia. To be more technical, to meet the criteria for schizoaffective disorder, the individual must experience either hallucinations or delusions for a 2-week period with no major mood symptoms of either depression or mania. At one time, the combination of lithium and haloperidol was commonly used to treat schizoaffective disorder. Today with the availability of atypical antipsychotic medications that block the dopamine receptors and serotonin receptors, monotherapy is an option. The combination medication Symbyax (fluoxetine plus olanzapine) is also an option as a blend of an SSRI and an atypical antipsychotic. The more traditional approach is an antipsychotic medication plus an antidepressant medication.

NONPHARMACOLOGIC TREATMENT APPROACHES FOR MOOD DISORDERS

Electroconvulsive Therapy

The treatment of psychiatric disorders includes several nonpharmacologic approaches that can be effective in treating mood disorders. Psychotherapy (see Chapter 13) has been the mainstay of psychiatry predating the use of medications. Another nonpharmacologic approach is the use of an electrical pulse to treat individuals. When psychotic individuals experienced a seizure due to abrupt discontinuation of their medications, their psychotic symptoms lessened. Because of this, physicians hypothesized that mental illness and seizure disorder could not coexist. This led to the concept of inducing seizures in individuals with mental illness as a form of treatment:

- In the 1500s, camphor-induced seizures were used to treat psychosis.
- In 1934 Ladislas J. von Meduna reintroduced the camphor technique by injecting it to induce seizures. He later switched from camphor to Metrazol (pentamethylenetetrazol). Von Meduna treated psychosis successfully in this manner from 1934 until 1938.
- In 1938 two psychiatrists in Rome, Italy, Ugo Cerletti and Lucio Bini, induced seizures with electrical pulse instead of the pentamethylenetetrazol injections. This technique was originally termed electroshock therapy and was later renamed electroconvulsive therapy (ECT).

Box 7. The Magic Number of 67

It is thought that if all of the current antidepressants available today were placed into a large container and all of the world's depressed individuals could walk by the container and reach in and take an antidepressant medication, 67% of individuals would improve on the medication. Schizophrenia seems to have the same 67% rate of success with antipsychotic medications. While this is a broad generalization and while the therapy must be carefully individualized, the result is that 33% of individuals with major depressive disorder and 33% of individuals with schizophrenia are often treatment resistant. The older studies of ECT show a treatment success rate of 75%, surpassing the benefit rate of medications. However, 3 reasons have relegated ECT to being the treatment approach used only after medication has proven ineffective:

1. Considerable stigma and many myths and misconceptions about ECT have resulted in strong social resistance to using ECT.
2. Many individuals experience temporary memory disruption and some individuals experience permanent memory disturbance after ECT.
3. Once performed, ECT cannot be undone.

The original dilemma with the electrically induced seizures was 2-fold. First, individuals expressed discomfort with the procedure. Second, many individuals experienced dental damage and bone fractures secondary to the muscle contractions during the seizure(s).

These 2 drawbacks were resolved by the medical ingenuity of the American psychiatrist Abram E. Bennett, who suggested anesthesia as a means of making the procedure safer and more tolerable. Succinylcholine became essential to the process. Today, ECT is performed in the surgical suite with the assistance of an anesthesiologist, often on an outpatient basis (Box 7).

No longer used solely for psychotic episodes, ECT is currently thought to be effective for a range of conditions, including:

- Primary uses
  - Major depressive disorder
  - Manic episodes/bipolar disorder
  - Schizophrenia, especially catatonic type
- Secondary uses
  - Delirium
  - Neuroleptic malignant syndrome
  - Obsessive-compulsive disorder
  - Parkinson's disease to treat the "on-off phenomenon"

ECT as Treatment – Major Depressive Disorder. For individuals who are acutely suicidal or homicidal, waiting 10 to 30 days for the medication to take effect may be unacceptable and unsafe. ECT can be used to immediately calm suicidal or homicidal ideations. It is also an effective treatment in the depressed individual who demonstrates agitation, stupor, and/or psychotic symptoms. As noted above, ECT is a reasonable option for individuals who fail to respond to antidepressant medications. If the ECT is also ineffective, these individuals may respond to a re-trial of antidepressant medications.

ECT as Treatment – Manic Episode/Bipolar Disorder. ECT is thought to be as effective as lithium in treating manic episodes. Because the current anti-manic medications have proven so effective, the use of ECT is most often reserved for those individuals who are acutely suicidal/homicidal, are unable to tolerate current medications, or have not achieved benefit from the current medications.

ECT as Treatment – Schizophrenia/Psychotic Episodes. ECT is thought to be effective for acute episodes of psychosis, yet not for the symptoms of chronic schizophrenia (see Chapter 3). ECT is thought to be dramatically effective in treating catatonia in schizophrenia.

The single most common side effect of ECT is disruption of memory, which usually resolves. Some individuals complain of persistent memory problems; in particular, in individuals for whom ECT is not effective, memory impairment may persist.

For individuals who are experiencing exacerbations of bipolar depression or mania during pregnancy, ECT is a safe alternative to reintroduction of the medications that may put both the fetus and mother at risk. While there are no absolute contraindications to ECT, one must be cautious if there are space-occupying lesions in the central nervous system. Individuals having had a recent myocardial infarction are also high-risk candidates; however, the risk is greatly diminished 2 weeks after the myocardial infarction and is even further decreased 3 months afterwards.

In performing ECT, the clinician can utilize either bilateral or unilateral placement of electrodes, as debate still exists as to which is more effective. In unilateral placement, both electrodes are placed over the nondominant hemisphere. In bilateral placement, an electrode is placed over each hemisphere. The number of ECT treatments varies, and is usually performed as 2 to 3 sessions per week. In major depressive disorder, anywhere from 6 to 12 treatments are used, with up to 20 sessions considered the maximum course. Manic episodes may require from 8 to 20 treatments. Schizophrenia may require at least 15 treatments, while catatonia and delirium may resolve in 1 to 4 treatments.

ECT is safe, effective, and treatment is usually time limited.

Repetitive Transcranial Magnetic Stimulation

Approved for use in the United States on October 8, 2008, this technique uses pulsed magnetic fields outside the individual's head. A small magnetic generator placed over the scalp at the prefrontal cortex generates a pulsed magnetic field by rapidly turning an electrical current on and off. This magnetic field depolarizes intracranial nerve cells impacting brain activity. Each rTMS session is performed without anesthesia, on an outpatient basis, and lasts approximately 15 to 30 minutes. Early studies used high-frequency electrical stimulation at 5 to 20 Hertz applied over the left prefrontal cortex. Recent research has shown effectiveness in treating depression with a lower frequency of 1 Hertz, applied to the right prefrontal cortex, with much less potential for a seizure than at the 5- to 20-Hertz level. At this point in time, it is thought that a individual must receive daily sessions for 3 weeks to achieve full benefit, given as 3 Monday through Friday series. The current FDA approval for this procedure is after an individual has had non-success with a pharmacologic approach.

Vagus Nerve Stimulation

Vagus nerve stimulation (VNS) was FDA approved for treating epilepsy in 1997, then for treating refractory depression in 2005. VNS requires the surgical implantation into the individual's chest of an electrical pacemaker device that stimulates the vagus nerve. Three electrical lead wires are connected to the vagus nerve in the left side of the neck. The exact mechanism of action is unknown. VNS and rTMS are thought to be alternatives to ECT.

THE FULL CIRCLE OF MOOD

Imagine mood as a clock (Figure 3). Euthymia, located at 12:00, represents the mood that most individuals call "fine." When they are "fine," they are balanced between the usual ranges of mood/emotion from happy to sad. Most individuals will comfortably and naturally move from euthymia to happy, from euthymia to sad, and back again.

- Those individuals who hover at 3 o'clock most of the day, every day, for at least 2 years meet the criteria for dysthymia. Dysthymia is a chronic low-level sadness that does not meet the criteria for a full-blown depressive episode.

- Those individuals who drop to 4 o'clock fall into depression. Depression is hallmarked by loss of interest in life activities and disruption in the neurovegetative functioning inventory indices of sleep, appetite, memory, concentration, energy, and libido. The depressed individual experiences a decrease in mood and may experience thoughts of wanting to die. The depressed individual experiences these life-disrupting feelings most of the day, every day, for at least 2 weeks.

- From euthymia, those individuals who cross gently beyond happy (9 o'clock) move into the mood level of hypomania (8 o'clock). In a hypomanic episode, the individual is a bit too effusive, just a bit too happy, and a bit too energetic. The hypomanic individual does not need as much sleep as usual, being much more work focused. Hypomania can prove constructive with the individual still able to work, function, and think coherently and competently.

- Individuals who fluctuate between dysthymia (3 o'clock) and hypomania (8 o'clock) suffer from a condition called cyclothymia. These individuals cycle between mildly decreased mood and mildly elevated mood. They are still functional in their daily lives.

- Individuals who go beyond hypomania and move into a mood too elevated or irritable, losing coherent, logical, reasonable thought, move into mania (7 o'clock). These individuals have distorted thinking, believing they are more important than they actually are (grandiosity), believing they can achieve and accomplish far beyond their actual potential, and going for days and nights without sleep.

- A full-blown manic episode in and of itself will qualify for the diagnosis of bipolar disorder type I. Once called manic-depressive, these are the classic bipolar individuals who experience both the highs and lows of the 2 poles. It is the extremes of the 2 poles that serve as the classic bipolar type I.

- The bipolar type II individual is the individual who has at least 1 episode of depression and at least 1 episode of hypomania.

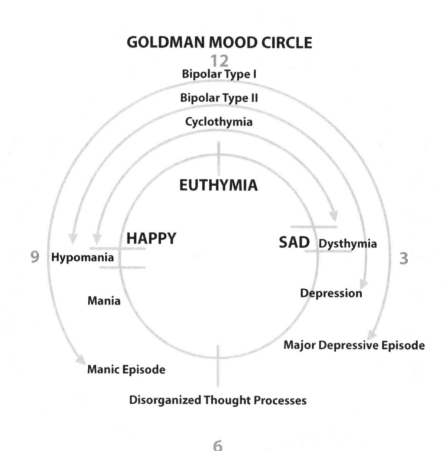

In the Goldman Mood Circle, Euthymia is the Center and serves as balanced mood.
The individual moves comfortably within the "normal" boundaries of Happy and Sad with Euthymia as the predominating state of being.
Cyclothymia = Cycling between Hypomania and Dysthymia
Bipolar Type I = At least one episode of Mania with or without alternating Depression
Bipolar Type II = Major Depressive Episode with at least one episode of Hypomania

Figure 3. The Goldman Mood Circle

The Goldman Guide to Psychiatry

CASE STUDY: MOOD DISORDERS

The individual, a 35-year-old white male, presents with the following symptoms that have been present most of the day, everyday, for at least two weeks:

- Decreased energy
- Decreased libido
- Decreased mood
- Frequent feelings of sadness and hopelessness
- Increased food consumption with a 25-pound weight gain over the past 2 months
- Memory and concentration less than premorbid levels
- Occasional thoughts of wanting to lie down and not wake up (passive suicidal ideations)
- Increased amount of sleep

The assessment process begins by asking first if the individual has any allergies to medications and documenting them prominently on the cover of the chart. Then the clinician asks the following series of questions:

- Have you ever suffered from these symptoms before?
- Were you placed on medication(s) previously?
- If so, which medications were prescribed?
- What dose was prescribed?
- Did the medication at that dose provide benefit?

The Diagnosis

This hypothetical individual has given the following information:

- Sleep disturbance (hypersomnolence)
- Appetite disturbance: increased eating with weight gain (hyperphagia)
- Memory below peak levels
- Concentration below peak levels
- Energy depleted (anergia)
- Libido decreased
- Suicidal (and homicidal) ideations: passive

The triad of hypersomnia, hyperphagia, and anergia leads to a diagnosis of atypical depression. The atypically depressed individual will also demonstrate mood reactivity with heightened sensitivity to social rejection. Atypical depression accounts for 42% to 48% of depressed individuals.

Therapeutic Considerations

In treating this individual with medications, the goal is to rebalance sleep, calm appetite, avoid disrupting memory or concentration, boost energy, and avoid further inhibition of libido. Once the depression is successfully treated, sleep, appetite, memory, concentration, energy, and libido should return to premorbid functioning.

TCAs, an older line medication approach, have a long history of success in treating depression. TCAs have the potential for anxiolysis (relief from anxiety), appetite stimulation and corresponding weight gain, and sedation, facilitating sleep at night and calming daytime anxiety and agitation. For the hypothetical individual, the side effects of sedation and weight gain make TCAs a poor choice, as the individual is already sleeping more than is appropriate and eating more than appropriate amounts of food. While the TCAs are less expensive than the newer line medications, they have significant potential for lethality in overdose. One TCA, Vivactil (protriptyline), is a possible option in treating atypical depression. Unlike other TCAs, protriptyline is activating instead of sedating; however, this potential for activation may exacerbate feelings of anxiousness.

The MAO inhibitors also have potential side effects of sedation and weight gain, making these medications unsuitable for the hypothetical individual.

The SSRIs are a reasonable option as a first-line treatment approach. While paroxetine has the potential for discontinuation syndrome, sedation, and weight gain, the SSRIs as a family have less potential for weight gain than the MAOIs or TCAs. They are also less sedating. When prescribing SSRIs remember to check sodium levels at least annually, as there is a possibility for sodium depletion (hyponatremia). They may also prolong clotting times.

Wellbutrin XL (bupropion) is primarily dopaminergic in its focus of action and is exquisitely tuned for treating atypical depression. Bupropion is noted to provide mild weight loss, improve energy, and enhance focus and concentration.

CHAPTER TWO

Anxiety Disorders

The concept of anxiety is relatively new in medicine. In 1871, Jacob Mendes DaCosta first described the condition in modern times in the *American Journal of Medical Sciences.* He gave this condition the label *irritable heart.* Noting the symptoms of chest pain, palpitations, and dizziness, he perceived the underlying cause to be an overactive nervous system adversely impacting the functioning of the heart. Using a soldier of the Civil War as his model, DaCosta observed anxiety and physical distress, congruent with the current diagnoses of acute stress disorder and post-traumatic stress disorder. He had discovered anxiety as the central core of the condition he labeled irritable heart.

Later, Sigmund Freud revisited the irritable heart concept and recognized the heart as an end organ being influenced by what he called *anxiety neurosis.*

Anxiety is analogous to hypertension. The body requires a level of intravascular pressure to move the nutrient-carrying blood throughout the system. Pressure must be maintained to carry blood to the brain and perfuse it continuously. Pressure must be adequate to carry away toxins and spent nutrients. The pressure must not become so high as to be dangerous to the integrity of the vessels themselves. Maintaining beneficial blood pressure is a normal function. When blood pressure goes awry and becomes too high, it becomes a health issue.

Similarly, a modicum of anxiety is productive. It gives the edge necessary to be successful and allows an individual to take work and its success seriously. Anxiety becomes problematic when this appropriate level becomes too great, anxiety with a capital "A." In mechanical terms, when the anxiety thermostat gets turned up too high, it becomes a health problem.

Some issues in anxiety can be identified as relating to a given anxiety-producing stimulus, others remain unclear. Acute stress disorder and post-traumatic stress disorder are related to a specific episode traumatizing the individual so powerfully that structural changes occur in the brain. These structural changes result in recurring memories of the episode. The underlying cause of panic disorder, on the other hand, is still unknown. The alerting system goes awry without provocation. The end result may be panic episodes.

Generalized anxiety disorder is similar to panic disorder in that the anxiety thermostat is turned up. However, in panic disorder, the individual experiences discrete attacks of red alert, whereas in generalized anxiety disorder, the increase in the anxiety thermostat moves moderately above usual and customary and remains constantly elevated on yellow alert.

Individuals with obsessive-compulsive disorder are thought to have a circuit disturbance in the brain that is analogous to the myocardial circuit disturbance of Wolf-Parkinson-White syndrome. In Wolf-Parkinson-White syndrome, there is a short-circuit in the electrical conduction through the myocardium, resulting in electrical looping of the cardiac impulse and causing a rapid cycling heart rate. In obsessive-compulsive disorder, the loop is thought to be between the frontal lobes, the basal ganglia, and the cingulum, resulting in a cycling and recycling of repetitive, intrusive thoughts.

CONCEPTUALIZING ANXIETY

To more clearly understand the anxiety disorders and the pharmacologic approaches to their treatment, one can categorize anxiety disorders based on the presence or absence of a known stressor and the degree of intrusion into the individual's day-to-day life:

- Anxiety due to a known psychosocial stressor
  - Social phobia
  - Acute stress disorder
  - Post-traumatic stress disorder
- Discrete anxiety (episodic occurrence of anxiety)
  - Panic disorder
  - Specific phobias
- Pervasive anxiety (no specific psychosocial stressor)
  - Agoraphobia
  - Generalized anxiety disorder
  - Obsessive-compulsive disorder
  - Social phobia

Anxiety Due to a Known Psychosocial Stressor

The anxiety disorders in this category have a readily identifiable psychosocial stressor at their core that generates the individual's discomfort.

Social Anxiety Disorder/Social Phobia. While social phobia may occur as a pervasive anxiety condition (see below), the condition also can be related to identifiable demands placed on the individual. In such instances, the individual's social phobia can be more specific in nature such as anxiousness at having to give presentations at the office or to attend office functions. The individual knows in which exact social situation(s) the discomfort occurs and the exact social stressor(s) that create(s) the anxious response. Nevertheless, the individual seems helpless to prevent the response.

Acute Stress Disorder. Acute stress disorder is the precursor, a "mini-version," of post-traumatic stress disorder. In acute stress disorder, the symptoms last a minimum of 2 days and a maximum of 30 days. If the symptoms persist beyond 30 days, the individual should be reassessed for post-traumatic stress disorder. In acute stress disorder, the underlying diagnostic criteria require individuals to have witnessed or experienced a life-threatening event, or perceived it to be such, resulting in intense fear, horror, or helplessness. These individuals must then experience any 3 of the following:

- A loss of awareness of their surrounding environment
- A loss of emotional responsiveness such as feeling detached or numb
- Feeling as if they are no longer themselves (depersonalization)
- Feeling as if they no longer exist in a real world (derealization)
- Shutting down their memory when they experience thoughts of the traumatic event (traumatic amnesia)

In combination with at least 3 of the above, individuals must also experience the traumatic event from 2 to 30 days in at least 1 of the following ways:

- Dreams of the trauma (nightmares)
- Reliving the traumatic event (revivification)
- Re-experiencing images of the trauma (flashbacks)
- Strong distress on being exposed to reminders of the event
- Thoughts of the trauma
- Visual cues misperceived as being the trauma (illusions)

The hallmarks of both acute stress disorder and post-traumatic stress disorder include:

- An increased level of arousal such that sleep and mood are disrupted
- Avoidance of any reminders of the traumatic event
- Disrupted concentration
- Ease to anger and irritability
- Exaggerated startle response
- Restlessness
- Traumatic paranoia, leading to hypervigilance to the surroundings

Post-Traumatic Stress Disorder. Post-traumatic stress disorder is to acute stress disorder as major depressive disorder is to adjustment disorder, with post-traumatic stress disorder being the more severe of the 2 trauma-induced anxiety disorders. As with acute stress disorder, individuals with post-traumatic stress disorder have experienced or witnessed a frightening event that has subjected them or someone within their visual field to the threat of serious physical injury or death. The individual must have also experienced intense fear or feeling of horror or helplessness. The diagnosis is confirmed when the individual also describes experiencing aspects of the following:

- **Reminders of the Event –** The individual continues to have recurrent, intrusive, distressing thoughts of the trauma either as dreams (nightmares), feeling as if the event were truly recurring (revivification), strong emotions, images (flashbacks), and/or thoughts. Reminders of the event create intense psychological distress and/or re-ignite physical responses to the event.

- **Avoidance of Reminders –** The individual seeks to avoid activities, conversations, feelings, places, thoughts, or people associated with the event. These individuals may also experience selective amnesia with regard to the traumatic event. The individual may lose interest in significant life activities, feel distanced from other people, or display a restricted range of affect. Finally, these individuals may sense feelings of doom or a fore-shortened future.

- **Increased Autonomic Response Since the Event –**After the traumatic event, the individual's autonomic nervous system has become over activated so that the individual may have difficulty falling asleep and/or staying asleep. The startle response is increased and traumatic paranoia may cause the individual to become hypervigilant to the surroundings. He or she may have a propensity to outbursts of anger and/or irritability or demonstrate disturbance in ability to focus and concentrate.

Discrete Anxiety
In this category of anxiety disorders, the individual demonstrates circumscribed types of anxiety in circumscribed episodic occurrences.

Panic Disorder. Panic disorder has as its hallmark the panic attack, which occurs suddenly and unexpectedly. The attack peaks within minutes and usually lasts from 5 minutes to as long as 30 minutes. While individuals may describe their panic attack as lasting for hours or days, what is probably occurring is a series of recurrent attacks/episodes, the persistence of residual generalized anxiety, or a more pervasive fear of having another attack (Box 1). The pervasive fear of having another attack, what one might call the *fear of fear itself*, is clinically called agoraphobia. Coming from the Greek word for *fear of the market place*, agoraphobia translates into the individual being afraid of being in an open setting, being away from a safe environment, and having an unexpected panic attack from which the individual can neither flee nor find comfort and support—hence the fear of fear itself.

Agoraphobia can lead the individual to become homebound and unable to go out into public. The panic attack results in dysregulation of the autonomic nervous system. The surge in the individual's physiologic anxiety thermostat results in:

- Physical symptoms
  - Changes in the body's perception of ambient temperature
  - Difficulty breathing
  - Feeling light headed
  - Increase in perspiration
  - Increase in heart rate
  - Nausea
  - Numbness and/or tingling in the extremities and/or face
  - Tightness in the throat
  - Tremulousness
  - Upset stomach

- Psychological symptoms
  - Feeling as if one is "going crazy"
  - Feeling detached from one's surroundings
  - Feeling detached from oneself (depersonalization)

Box 1: Goldman's Theory of Status Panicus

Many individuals describe a panic attack as lasting several hours or even all day. What the individual is actually experiencing is a discrete panic attack followed by agoraphobia that leads into another attack. This cycle may repeat itself all day, a condition that could be called *status panicus*. This is the anxiety analogue of status epilepticus, in which the individual experiences the seizure episode as recurring over and over without remission. The period immediately following an epileptic seizure is known as the post-ictal phase. In this phase, individuals have a clouded sensorium as they slowly return to full awareness and consciousness. When individuals experience several seizure episodes in succession, individuals will experience an inter-ictal phase, a period between seizures with continued clouded sensorium. Similarly, in panic disorder, the individual may experience an aura, a presage of the onset of the panic attack, followed by the panic attack itself. Once the initial panic attack has subsided, the individual experiences a feeling of discomfort and the fear of another panic attack onset. The period after a panic attack can be post-ictal, meaning *after the thing*, and the period between panic attacks as inter-ictal, meaning *between the things*, as analogous to the same episodes in epileptic seizures. This fear of the onset of another panic attack is the post-ictal or inter-ictal agoraphobia, which leads to another panic attack. This may repeat itself multiple times throughout the day. Thus, the individual is experiencing:

- An initial feeling of uneasiness (the **panic attack aura**)→ THE PANIC ATTACK
- THE PANIC ATTACK→ uneasiness and the fear of another attack (POST-ICTAL AGORAPHOBIA)
- POST-ICTAL AGORAPHOBIA→onset of another **panic attack**
- PANIC ATTACK→ POST-ICTAL AGORAPHOBIA
- POST-ICTAL AGORAPHOBIA→onset of another **panic attack**
- The sum of the above is STATUS PANICUS

The Goldman Guide to Psychiatry

- Feeling of impending doom or of dying
- Feeling unreal (derealization)

Individuals meet the diagnostic criteria for panic disorder if they experience any 4 of the above symptoms and at least 1 month (or more) of continuing concern about having another attack; changing significantly their behavior related to the attacks; or what the implications of having an attack could be.

Comorbid psychiatric conditions often found with panic disorder are major depressive disorder and substance abuse. Because of the recurrent, unexpected frightening episodes of panic attacks, it is not uncommon for individuals to become depressed and feel that life is not worth living. Many individuals will seek to self-medicate with legal substances such as alcohol and tobacco, and numerous illicit substances. Some individuals may be at risk for suicide.

To ensure an accurate diagnosis, the clinician should rule out medical disorders that present with signs and symptoms similar to panic disorder, including:

- Diseases of the vestibular nerve
- Hyperparathyroidism
- Hyperthyroidism
- Hypoglycemia
- Pheochromocytoma
- Supraventricular tachycardia

The clinician should also ask about the use and/or abuse of caffeine. Hyper-caffeinism mimics a panic attack. High consumption levels of coffee, cola beverages, and chocolate containing varying amounts of caffeine may be the culprit for many of the symptoms perceived as a panic attack.

Specific Phobias. Fear is often an appropriate and adaptive response to specific situations that are dangerous. Fear, like pain, is a signal alerting us to either act or cease from engaging in a specific activity or situation. Some fears, however, can become inappropriate, excessive, and counter-productive. Fear is termed a phobia when it is disproportionate to the real danger or discomfort caused by ideas, objects, places, and situations.

There are 3 main phobias in the psychiatric setting:

- Agoraphobia: The *fear of fear itself.* This is the fear that one will have a fearful episode or an attack with no means of escaping to a safe place.

- Social anxiety disorder/social phobia: The fear of participating in generalized or specific social activities or events. This is shyness taken to its discomforting extreme.
- Specific phobia: The fear of an object, idea, situation or specific place.

Specific phobias are thought to affect 25% to 33% of the American population. These fears, however, bring individuals into the psychiatrist's office much less often than other disorders. Estimates are that 1 in 10 individuals present to a psychiatrist's office with obsessive-compulsive disorder, while only 2 to 3 of 100 present because of a specific phobia. The most common specific phobias bringing individuals to the psychiatrist's office are fear of driving over bridges, fear of flying, and fear of riding in elevators or on escalators. These fears stand out because they impede the individual's daily activities. Fear of rodents, snakes, or spiders is manageable for most people by avoiding the stimulus of their fears. Driving, flying, and riding in elevators and on escalators, on the other hand, are not easily avoided in today's busy world. Most individuals with specific phobias will comprehend intellectually that their fear is irrational.

Pervasive Anxiety
In this category of anxiety disorders, the feeling of anxiousness is neither discrete nor time-limited. Individuals experience the dread of anxiety most of the day and night almost every day and night of their lives.

Agoraphobia. As noted above, agoraphobia is the fear of fear itself. This is the fear of being away from a safe environment and having an unexpected panic attack from which the individual cannot flee or find comfort and support. Agoraphobia is most often associated with panic attacks; however, it can occur on its own, without the panic attacks actually happening. It is the overpowering fear of having a panic attack that can prove absolutely debilitating for these individuals, causing them to be afraid to leave their homes.

Generalized Anxiety Disorder. The prototype of the pervasive occurrence of anxiety, generalized anxiety disorder is a constant uneasy feeling about life. It is an excessive state of worry that is difficult for the individual to control, the proverbial waiting for the other shoe to fall. Generalized anxiety disorder differs from panic disorder in that the individual has an increase in the anxiety thermostat so that it is moderately elevated almost all of the time. In other words, panic disorder is discrete episodes of red alert, while generalized anxiety disorder is best described as the individual always being on yellow alert. The diagnosis requires that the individual experience for most of the day, every day for at least 6 months, 3 or more of the following symptoms:

- Difficulty in falling asleep or maintaining sleep, or awakening unrefreshed
- Easily angered or irritated
- Feeling edgy or restless
- Feeling fatigued
- Feeling vague somatic discomfort such as muscle tension

Social Anxiety Disorder/Social Phobia. Social phobia can occur as a discrete episode or pervasively affect the individual's entire life. This is the fear of being humiliated or embarrassed in a public setting. Unlike agoraphobia, this is not the fear of being away from home and having a panic attack. Instead, the fear comes from knowing that the social event itself will cause the anxiousness. This may be as specific as fear of public speaking, fear of eating in a public restaurant, or fear of using a public restroom (sometimes referred to as shy bladder). In its pervasive form, the individual feels extremely uncomfortable interacting with others, including yet not limited to interacting with work colleagues, making conversation at a party, or being present in a large crowd. Social phobia occurs as both a pervasive anxiety phenomenon and as a discrete anxiety disorder due to a known psychosocial stressor. It is thought that social phobia begins in adolescence.

Obsessive-Compulsive Disorder. French psychiatrist Jean Etienne Esquirol first described obsessive-compulsive disorder as an illness in 1838 in his treatise *Des Maladies Mentales*. Obsessive-compulsive disorder was originally categorized as a depressive illness. Then Sigmund Freud applied his concept of intrapsychic conflict to this disorder, generating his label of obsessional neurosis. As psychiatry began shifting into the biological model, Freud's obsessional neurosis was renamed obsessive-compulsive disorder in 1980.

While the definitive etiology of obsessive-compulsive disorder is still unknown, findings from the newest scanning technologies have demonstrated increased glucose metabolism in the caudate nuclei of the basal ganglia, the cingulum, and the orbital cortex of the frontal lobes. The scans show partial normalization after treatment with serotonergic medications such as Anafranil (clomipramine) and the serotonin selective reuptake inhibitors (SSRIs). The disorder appears to have a strong genetic component as well.

In 1999, Susan E. Swedo of the National Institute of Mental Health described cases of sudden onset of obsessive-compulsive disorder with motor tics, mood lability, and separation anxiety in children and adolescents aged 9 to 15 years after they experienced a group A beta hemolytic streptococcal infection. This syndrome was given the acronym of PANDAS for **P**ediatric **A**utoimmune **N**eurologic **D**isorder **A**fter **S**treptococcal infection. This suggests there may be a bacterial and/or viral etiology for some of the obsessive-compulsive disorder cases seen.

An estimated 1 in 10 individuals visiting an outpatient psychiatrist's office presents because of obsessive-compulsive disorder. The following are common types of presentation:

1. Thoughts of being contaminated by germs and/or dirt; the individual feels, "I must wash my hands!"
2. Thoughts of self-doubt; the individual asks himself or herself, "Did I lock the front door? Did I turn off the coffee pot? Was the pothole I just ran over a person instead?"
3. Thoughts of symmetry; the individual's self-talk includes, "My shoes must all face the same direction! All my shirts/blouses must hang in the closet in the same way! My desk must be clean before I leave the office for the day!"
4. Thoughts of needing to keep items because of overvaluing them; the individual engages in hoarding, "I must keep this newspaper as someday I will need to refer to the front page!"

As summarized in Table 1, the corresponding actions (compulsions) in which the individual engages to release the anxiety caused by the above thoughts (obsessions) are, in corresponding order:

1. Washing and/or cleaning; avoiding certain objects, places, or persons
2. Checking locks or appliances; confessing errors/mistakes; asking forgiveness
3. Organizing and arranging in a given manner; repetitive counting
4. Hoarding/saving

Table 1. Common Obsessions and Their Corresponding Compulsions

Thought (Obsession)	Action (Compulsion)
Fear of germs	Washing/cleaning
Doubt	Checking/confessing
Symmetry	Organizing
Object value	Hoarding

PRESCRIBING MEDICATIONS FOR ANXIETY DISORDERS: CLINICAL TIPS AND PEARLS

Note: Before initiating any therapy, the clinician should obtain informed consent from the individual, parent, or guardian (see Appendix 1).

As described above, anxiety is manifested as different types that range from pervasive anxiousness to discrete episodes. The specific type of anxiety determines the focus of the pharmacologic approach (Table 2).

Table 2. Current SSRIs FDA Approved for Treating Anxiety Disorders

Medications	Generalized Anxiety Disorder	Obsessive-Compulsive Disorder	Panic Disorder	Post-Traumatic Stress Disorder	Social Phobia
Effexor XR (venlafaxine)	Yes		Yes		Yes
Lexapro (escitalopram)	Yes				
Luvox (fluvoxamine)		Yes			Yes
Paxil (paroxetine)	Yes	Yes	Yes	Yes	Yes
Prozac (fluoxetine)		Yes	Yes		
Zoloft (sertraline)		Yes	Yes	Yes	Yes

Panic Disorder

Panic attacks are frightening and debilitating. Individuals fear they are dying. They experience a multitude of distressing physical symptoms, including yet not limited to chest tightness, choking sensation, heart palpitations, lightheadedness, nausea, perspiration, shakiness and tremulousness, and shortness of breath.

As discussed, the panic attack may generate the agoraphobic fear of having another panic attack, the fear of being in a place from which there is no timely and safe exit. It is this agoraphobia that may ultimately lead individuals to becoming homebound. Cognitive and behavioral therapeutic approaches assist in providing relief. Intervening with medication may be the pivotal therapy. By calming the acute psychiatric fever, medication allows the individual to realize that life is not ending, and he or she is able to actively participate in psychotherapy. The pharmacologic approaches are as follows:

- Antipsychotic medications (the atypicals)
- Benzodiazepines
- Buspar (buspirone)
- Effexor XR (venlafaxine)
- Gamma-amino butyric acid (GABA)-ergic medications
- Inderal (propranolol)
- Monoamine oxidase (MAO) inhibitors
- Nefazodone
- SSRIs
- Tricyclic antidepressants

Atypical Antipsychotic Medications. Currently, atypical antipsychotic medications are being used off-label to calm anxiety. Risperdal (risperidone) and Seroquel (quetiapine) are most commonly used in small doses. Risperidone is dosed at 0.25 mg by mouth 1 to 4 times per day and quetiapine is dosed at 25 mg by mouth 1 to 4 times per day.

Benzodiazepines. These medications offer the most immediate relief from the power of the panic attack. However, the clinician should be cautious and maintain an index of suspicion for the risk of tolerance and dependence. Tolerance manifests when the individual becomes less responsive to a particular medication dose over time. Dependence necessitates the continued administration of the medication to prevent the appearance of withdrawal symptoms. For panic disorder, 3 benzodiazepines are commonly used:

- **Ativan (lorazepam)** is clinically slower to onset and offset than another benzodiazepine Xanax (alprazolam) and is better to prophylactically avoid or avert a panic attack. Lorazepam has the potential for dependency if used on a long-term basis, and caution should be used if both nefazodone and lorazepam are prescribed simultaneously. Lorazepam is prescribed at 0.25 to 0.5 mg to calm a panic attack and prophylactically at 0.25 to 0.5 mg 2 to 4 times a day. If used daily for greater than 2 to 3 weeks, lorazepam should not be abruptly discontinued because of the potential for discontinuation (withdrawal) seizures.

- **Klonopin (clonazepam)** demonstrates the longest benefit per dose of the 3 most popular medications in this category. Clinically, it is slower to onset and offset than lorazepam, giving clonazepam the greatest potential for scheduled dosing for prophylaxis of panic attacks. As a prophylactic or maintenance dose, clonazepam is prescribed at 0.5 to 1 mg by mouth once in the morning and again in early evening (5 to 7 PM). Some clinicians will prescribe it 3 times per day, so the individual receives 0.5 to 1 mg first in the morning, then again at midafternoon and the last dose just before bedtime. Some individuals need the bedtime dose to prevent the onset of a panic attack during the night and early morning. Clonazepam should not be abruptly discontinued because of the potential for discontinuation (withdrawal) seizures.

- **Xanax (alprazolam)** provides rapid onset of benefit. The dose may be as low as 0.25 mg by mouth when an episode occurs or prophylactically as 0.25 mg by mouth 2 to 4 times a day. Some individuals may need to increase the dose amount. Whenever possible, it is prudent to use alprazolam on an as-needed basis, as it can lead to tolerance and dependence if used long term. When possible, alprazolam should be prescribed concurrently as the clinician initiates therapy with an SSRI, Buspar (buspirone), or a tricyclic antidepressant, with the goal to discontinue alprazolam once the other medication is effective. Caution should be used when prescribing alprazolam at the same time as nefazodone, as the potency of alprazolam is quadrupled by nefazodone. A newer delivery formulation (Niravam) can be taken without water. If used daily for greater than 2 to 3 weeks, alprazolam should not be abruptly discontinued because of the potential for discontinuation (withdrawal) seizures.

Some individuals with panic disorders will not receive benefit from any medication other than the benzodiazepines. When prescribing a benzodiazepine, the clinician should be forthright about the potential for tolerance and dependence. If the individual begins to increase the amount of an individual dose or the number of times during the day that each dose is being taken, the clinician should suspect tolerance is occurring and formulate a new treatment plan.

Buspar (buspirone). Buspirone can take from 2 to 6 weeks to demonstrate benefit. It is often initiated concomitantly with a benzodiazepine, in which case as the individual approaches the second week of taking buspirone, the benzodiazepine is discontinued and the individual is maintained solely on buspirone. For individuals who are medication naïve, that is, they have not taken a previous medication for panic disorder, buspirone can prove beneficial. Individuals who have had a longstanding history of using a benzodiazepine medication may get little benefit from buspirone. The medication often proves more beneficial for generalized anxiety disorder, for which it is approved by the US Food and Drug Administration (FDA), than for panic disorder.

Effexor XR (venlafaxine). Venlafaxine has been used at low doses (37.5 mg by mouth each day) to help relieve panic attacks and anxiety. It is beneficial for generalized anxiety disorder or anxiety with depression/depression with anxiety. It is FDA approved for generalized anxiety disorder, panic disorder, and social anxiety disorder/social phobia.

GABA-ergic Medications. This group of medications, including Gabitril (tiagabine) and Neurontin (gabapentin), has demonstrated effectiveness in treating anxiety off-label. These 2 medications are antiseizure medications that enhance the postsynaptic availability of GABA. It is thought that greater availability of postsynaptic GABA produces a calming effect. Lyrica (pregabalin) is a GABA analogue currently approved to treat diabetic neuropathic pain, fibromyalgia, and post-herpetic neuralgia, and as an adjunctive treatment for partial seizures. It is currently being used off-label to treat generalized anxiety disorder.

Inderal (propranolol). Propranolol is a beta-blocker that is used for treating hypertension, prophylactically for migraine headaches, and off-label for treating generalized anxiety disorder. For individuals with occasional panic attacks, propranolol is an off-label option. It is also prescribed for performance anxiety and used by actors/actresses, musicians, speakers, and other performers who cannot tolerate cognitive dulling or motor function disturbance that may result from benzodiazepine use.

MAO Inhibitors. MAO inhibitors have been shown to be effective in treating panic disorder. When prescribed MAO inhibitors, individuals must avoid foods and liquids that contain tyramine. Combining tyramine with an MAO inhibitor creates the potential for an hypertensive crisis. The MAO inhibitors also do not mix well with other medications, including alternative supplements. St. John's wort, a popular "natural" antidepressant and anxiolytic that is available in health food stores, is thought to have MAO inhibitor qualities.

Nefazodone. Used off-label, nefazodone may provide benefit for some individuals with panic disorder, generalized anxiety disorder, or stress-related anxiety, although it is most beneficial for treating major depressive disorder with an anxious component. Dosing this medication 3 to 4 times a day in 25-mg to 50-mg doses provides benefit for many anxious individuals. When prescribing nefazodone, clinicians should:

- Advise individuals of a possible LSD-like side effect, palinopsia. Palinopsia, also referred to as visual trailing, is the continued visual perception of an image after the stimulus for the image has left the visual field.
- Allow for a 2- to 4-week washout of an SSRI before initiating nefazodone because of the metabolite mCPP.
- Allow for a 2-week washout from nefazodone before initiating an SSRI.

SSRIs. The SSRIs may provide relief from panic attacks over time. In the first 2 weeks of treatment with an SSRI, the individual may experience some jitteriness, which may be misinterpreted as anxiety.

When utilizing an SSRI to treat an anxiety disorder, it is recommended to initiate with a low dose and slowly titrate upward as clinically indicated.

- Celexa (citalopram) is initiated at 10 mg and its enantiomer cousin, Lexapro (escitalopram), is initiated at 2.5 to 5mg by mouth each day. Escitalopram is FDA approved for treating generalized anxiety disorder.
- Luvox CR (fluvoxamine maleate) is initiated at 100mg by mouth each day (for OCD and Social phobia) and titrated upward as clinically indicated.
- Paxil (paroxetine) is initiated at 5 mg by mouth each day and titrated upward as clinically indicated. Paroxetine is FDA approved for generalized anxiety disorder, obsessive-compulsive disorder, panic disorder, post-traumatic stress disorder, and social anxiety disorder. A controlled-release formula is FDA approved for panic disorder. It is initiated at 12.5 mg per day.
- Prozac (fluoxetine) is initiated at 5 to 10 mg by mouth either every other day or every day, depending on effectiveness.
- Zoloft (sertraline) is initiated at 12.5 mg by mouth each day.

Tricyclic Antidepressants (TCAs). TCAs provide benefit for treating panic attacks and anxiety, although they may need 2 to 3 weeks before demonstrating benefit. Sometimes TCAs will initially exacerbate the attacks. TCAs also improve underlying or concomitant depression. Tofranil (imipramine) and Anafranil (clomipramine) are effective in children and adults. Clomipramine has the added advantage of being effective for obsessive-compulsive disorder because of the medication's serotonergic reuptake inhibition. Individuals experiencing panic attacks report the greatest effectiveness when the doses are split into 2 or 3 times a day. The medication's mildly sedating quality helps to calm the fear of a recurring attack.

Generalized Anxiety Disorder

Individuals with generalized anxiety disorder experience the persistent phenomenon of waiting for the other shoe to fall. A variety of pharmacologic treatment approaches, on and off-label, are available.

Atypical Antipsychotic Medications. The atypical antipsychotics are often used off-label to treat anxiety, especially generalized anxiety disorder. While aripiprazole is FDA approved as adjunctive therapy in treating major depressive disorder, it is not approved for use in anxiety disorders and is not typically used to treat anxiety disorders.

Benzodiazepines. Benzodiazepines have rapid onset of benefit. Because abrupt discontinuation after 3 to 4 weeks of steady use can result in a withdrawal seizure, tapering to discontinuation is advised.

Buspirone. Buspirone works as an agonist or partial agonist at the serotonin ($5HT_{1A}$) receptor site. Unlike the benzodiazepines, it does not act on the GABA channels, nor does it have the abuse potential of the benzodiazepines. By the same token, it does not have their rapid onset of benefit either; it may take from 2 to 6 weeks for buspirone to display benefit. The medication needs to be taken every day, not on an as-needed basis, and it must be taken several times a day. It can be initiated at 5 mg by mouth 2 to 3 times a day and may be increased to 10 mg 2 to 3 times a day. Some individuals may need to take as much as 20 mg 3 times a day at its maximum dosing range. If an individual has been on a benzodiazepine for a long time and needs to change medications, one option is to initiate buspirone as the benzodiazepine is slowly tapered to discontinuation. Unfortunately, for some individuals who are used to the immediate onset of benefit from benzodiazepines, switching to buspirone may prove somewhat unfulfilling. Nevertheless, it is worth a trial.

Clonidine. Clonidine is an alpha$_2$ agonist that was originally developed for treating hypertension. It is used off-label for treating anxiety related to general anxiety disorder or post-traumatic stress disorder. While the medication helps calm nightmares for many individuals, it can paradoxically cause nightmares in others.

MAO Inhibitors. The MAO inhibitors offer some benefit for relieving anxiety. Because of side effects, the potential for med-med interactions, and reaction with tyramine-containing foods, the MAO inhibitors have typically been initiated as a second-line approach. With the advent of the transdermal patch delivery system for Emsam (selegiline), MAO inhibitors are once again considered first-line approach therapy for anxiety. The transdermal patch delivery system circumvents the first-pass effect, so it is thought that at low dose (6mg), taking Emsam (selegiline) avoids the oral MAO inhibitors' dietary risks.

Nefazodone. Nefazodone is a second-generation SSRI. Because of its 5HT$_2$ receptor blockade, it serves to improve mood and calm anxiety. By blocking the 5HT$_2$ receptor, this medication calms jitteriness and minimizes the side effects of insomnia and sexual dysfunction. Due to the potential for acute hepatotoxicity, this is no longer used first-line.

Propranolol. Propranolol is a beta-blocker that was developed for treating hypertension and is used off-label for treating anxiety. It has shown greatest effectiveness in calming generalized anxiety disorder and social anxiety disorder/social phobia. It is dosed at 10 to 20 mg before the anxiety-provoking event for social anxiety disorder, or 10 to 20 mg 2 to 3 times a day for generalized anxiety disorder.

SSRI Antidepressants. SSRIs show benefit at low doses for calming anxiety. While their primary benefit is for treating depression, some are FDA approved for different types of anxiety. In particular, escitalopram and paroxetine are FDA approved for treating generalized anxiety disorder.

TCAs. TCAs have the primary benefit of treating depression. They also help calm anxiety and have proven to be effective for generalized anxiety disorder.

Venlafaxine. Venlafaxine is FDA approved for treating generalized anxiety disorder, as well as social anxiety disorder/social phobia and panic disorder. For calming generalized anxiety disorder, the medication is initiated at 37.5 mg for 7 to 10 days and then reassessed. Some individuals will need an increase to 75 mg, while others may need to go as high as 150 mg to calm their generalized anxiety disorder. Note, these doses refer to the extended release (XR) formulation.

Social Anxiety Disorder/Social Phobia

Propranolol can be used at 10 mg by mouth approximately an hour before an anxiety-producing social situation or dosed at 20 mg, if needed. Some individuals have found propranolol to be effective when dosed 2 or 3 times a day for social phobia and performance anxiety. Clinicians should monitor the individual's blood pressure during the dose-titration process.

Fluvoxamine, paroxetine, sertraline, and venlafaxine are FDA approved for treating social phobia. The MAO inhibitor Nardil (phenelzine) also shows benefit.

Obsessive-Compulsive Disorder

Obsessive-compulsive disorder is typically a life-long condition, for which medication will provide varying levels of relief. Medications that focus on the neurotransmitter of serotonin have proven to be most effective in treating obsessive-compulsive disorder. The medications that are FDA approved are the TCA clomipramine and the SSRIs fluoxetine, fluvoxamine, paroxetine, and sertraline.

Treating obsessive-compulsive disorder with SSRIs typically requires prescribing at the high end of their dosing range. The regimen starts the SSRI at the low end, allowing an assessment for tolerability and monitoring for side effects. Then, assuming no negative effects are found, the individual can increase the medication at a comfortable rate.

- For clomipramine, the maximum dose per day is 250 mg. The medication has the potential to lower the seizure threshold, as do so many of the psychotropic medications, so caution is warranted at higher doses (eg, 200 mg per day), due to the seizure potential. Individuals with prior head trauma, in particular, must be closely monitored. It is initiated at bedtime because of its sedating quality.

- Escitalopram can be dosed to 30 or 40 mg as tolerated. While it is not currently FDA approved for treating obsessive-compulsive disorder, many clinicians find it effective.

- Fluoxetine is dosed up to 60 to 80 mg per day.

- Fluvoxamine will be most effective when dosed at 200 mg to 300 mg per day, most often in a divided twice-a-day dosing schedule. Fluvoxamine should not be prescribed concurrently with theophylline. Luvox CR (fluvoxamine maleate) was FDA approved on February 28, 2008 for treating OCD (and social phobia).

- Paroxetine is typically titrated to 40 to 60mg per day to achieve its greatest effectiveness for treating OCD.

- Sertraline is often titrated to its maximum package insert dose of 200 mg per day for treating OCD.

It can take up to 3 months for medications to provide benefit for individuals with obsessive-compulsive disorder. In addition, individuals will receive differing levels of benefit, all idiosyncratic based on the individual. Some individuals will achieve 100% relief, while others may only achieve 10% to 25% benefit. Furthermore, obsessive-compulsive disorder seems to go through exacerbations and remissions. One medication may work well for a while and then it may tend to poop out, at which point the clinician can:

- Increase the dose
- Augment with another medication, particularly the benzodiazepine clonazepam
- Change to another medication altogether

Once a medication achieves effectiveness, the clinician should stress continued compliance. If the individual misses doses or discontinues the medication, it will often no longer prove as effective when it is re-initiated. Therapy for obsessive-compulsive disorder is equivalent to balancing on a tightrope. Once effectiveness of a medication is achieved, it is important not to vary the dosing or the timing.

The medications FDA approved for treating obsessive-compulsive disorder in children and adolescents are clomipramine, fluoxetine, fluvoxamine, and sertraline.

Post-Traumatic Stress Disorder

Post-traumatic stress disorder is treated with both psychotherapy (see Chapter 13) and medication. Four prescription medications have shown benefit:

Clonidine. An alpha$_2$ agonist, clonidine may be dosed starting with 0.05 to 0.1 mg at bedtime and may be titrated upward to multiple doses (2 to 4 times) throughout the day, not to exceed 0.4 mg per day in total. Blood pressure should be monitored to avoid hypotension. While clonidine is given to calm autonomic nervous system responses and to inhibit nightmares, paradoxically it may cause nightmares in some people, which should be monitored. Also, this medication should not be stopped abruptly, as rebounding hypertension can result.

Paroxetine. This SSRI medication is FDA approved for treating post-traumatic stress disorder. Dosing of the immediate-release form begins at 10 mg with upward titration to 20 or 30 mg per day. The continuous release form, Paxil CR (paroxetine hydrochloride CR), is usually initiated at 12.5 mg per day and titrated upward to 37.5 mg per day.

Sertraline. This SSRI is FDA approved for treating post-traumatic stress disorder. The medication is initiated at 12.5 mg by mouth for 4 to 6 days and then increased to 25 mg. If the individual has not achieved benefit after 7 days at 25 mg, the medication is titrated upward to benefit in 25-mg to 50-mg increments every 2 weeks. The current package insert maximum dosing is 200 mg per day.

Sinequan (doxepin). This TCA calms anxiety, improves mood, and suppresses nightmares. It is typically initiated as 25 mg by mouth at bedtime and titrated upward by 25 mg to an effective dose, not exceeding 300 mg per day. If it is not effective by 100 to 150 mg, the clinician is advised to taper downward and seek another medication. As a TCA, doxepin has the potential to cause blurred vision, constipation, dry mouth, sedation, slowing electrical conduction through the heart, urinary retention, weight gain and lethality in overdose. The urinary retention effect can be a serious issue for older men who have benign prostatic hypertrophy. Clinicians should inquire about an individual's nighttime bladder habits and evaluate for benign prostatic hypertrophy in male individuals. If the diagnosis is confirmed, doxepin should not be prescribed.

CHAPTER THREE

Thought Disorders

Psychosis is the disorganization of thoughts. Individuals suffering from psychotic episodes demonstrate strange behaviors that are the result of strange thought processes. Put simply, strange thoughts cause strange behaviors.

While all strange behaviors are not necessarily due to strange thoughts, strange thoughts will often beget strange/odd behaviors. Typically, odd thoughts are the filter through which the individual sees the world. These thoughts are shaped by disturbances in what one thinks one hears (auditory hallucinations), sees (visual hallucinations), and/or feels (tactile hallucinations). Psychotic individuals may be free from any hallucinations and suffer instead from a fixed, false belief, known as a delusion, about what is going on in their lives. Historically, medical doctrine was that psychotic episodes did not occur until a person had reached late adolescence or early adulthood. For reasons unknown, young children now present with psychotic episodes.

DELUSIONAL DISORDER

An individual with a circumscribed fixed, false belief of a non-bizarre nature suffers from delusional disorder. A non-bizarre delusion is a thought disturbance focusing on a realistic situation that can occur in life, such as being:

- Deceived by a spouse or lover
- Followed or stalked
- Infected by a disease
- Loved at a distance
- Poisoned

An individual suffering from delusional disorder typically goes about each day as if nothing is out of order except for the circumscribed delusional process. These individuals may still go to work and function appropriately; they may still participate in social activities, except for those related to the circumscribed special idiosyncrasy. Along with eating disorders (which often have a delusional component), delusional disorder is one of the most difficult psychiatric conditions to successfully treat.

SCHIZOPHRENIA

Schizophrenia is found in all cultures and has a worldwide prevalence of 1% of the population. This disease typically has its first onset in late adolescence (ages 17 to 21 years) or early adulthood. Because schizophrenia occurs just as the young person is entering adulthood, the disease proves particularly devastating.

Schizophrenia's Historical Perspective

- In 1851 Jean Pierre Falret wrote of a cyclic madness he called *folie circulair* (actually describing the phenomena of what were later termed *cyclothymia and bipolar disorder*).
- In 1871, Ewald Hecker wrote about hebephrenia, which he named in honor of the goddess of youth and frivolity (Hebe), because he viewed the individual as silly and demonstrating a frivolous mind.
- In 1874, Karl Ludwig Kahlbaum described a movement disorder with statue-like stiffness of the muscles and odd postures, catatonia, combined with an incredible sense of fear, paranoia.
- In 1878, Emil Kraepelin presented the term *dementia praecox* to the world. Kraepelin observed that the individuals demonstrated an early onset (praecox) of a progressive deterioration and disruption of cognitive function (dementia).
- In 1911, Eugen Bleuler introduced the concept of schizophrenia. Bleuler did not share Kraepelin's perception of a global dementing process. Instead he believed that the mind was split between what the individual was feeling subjectively and what the individual manifested as the corresponding thoughts. Bleuler described 4 components of this division of mind and feelings with his famous 4 A's:
  - Affect manifested as a diminished emotional response to external and internal stimuli; the individual appeared emotionally blunted.
  - Ambivalence referred to difficulty in decision-making. The individual's awareness of the surrounding environment disintegrated and with it came the inability to process incoming information.
  - Associations of thoughts became loosened, making the individual's thinking appear odd and disorganized.
  - Autism was the state in which individuals withdrew from the world around them, drawing ever more closely inward.

In addition, Bleuler categorized schizophrenia into 4 types:
  - Catatonic schizophrenia, presenting with the lack of expression and movement.
  - Hebephrenic schizophrenia, presenting as disordered motor movement.

- Paranoid schizophrenia, presenting as fear and thoughts of being persecuted.
- Simple schizophrenia, presenting as the slow progressive loss of social function with withdrawal and apathy.

Modern Concept of Schizophrenia

In 1959 Kurt Schneider introduced the concept of "first rank" symptoms for schizophrenia. His criteria set the foundation for the *Diagnostic and Statistical Manual of Mental Disorders, 4th Edition-TR* diagnosis for schizophrenia. To meet the criteria for the diagnosis of schizophrenia, the individual must experience 1 of the following primary criteria:

- Suffer from bizarre delusions
- Hear voices that either maintain a running commentary of the individual's thoughts or have 2 or more voices conversing with each other

If individuals do not suffer from either of these primary criteria, then they must experience at least 2 of the following:

- Delusions
- Disorganized behavior or catatonia
- Disorganized speech
- Hallucinations
- Symptoms similar to Bleuler's 4 A's presenting as affective flattening, decrease in speech, decline in motivation, and/or withdrawal inward

The individual must also have a disturbance in social, occupational, or hygiene function from the onset of the illness. Finally, to be diagnosed as schizophrenia, the symptoms must have persisted beyond 6 months' duration.

Box 1. Brief Psychotic Disorder vs. Schizophreniform Disorder vs. Schizophrenia

- Brief psychotic disorder is the diagnosis applied to a disturbance in thought lasting from 1 to 30 days.
- Schizophreniform disorder is the diagnosis applied to a thought disturbance persisting beyond 30 days and resolving within 6 months.
- Schizophrenia is diagnosed when the thought disturbance persists beyond 6 months.

Current psychiatric dogma delineates 5 subtypes of schizophrenia:

- Catatonic – The individual demonstrates 2 or more of the following:
  - Catalepsy with waxy flexibility or stupor
  - Echolalia or echopraxia
  - Increased motor activity (referred to as catatonic excitement)
  - Mutism
  - Odd posturing or stereotyped movements
- Disorganized – The individual displays disorganization of speech or behavior, a flattening of affect, or inappropriate affect.
- Paranoid – The individual suffers from auditory hallucinations or delusions.
- Residual – The individual's schizophrenic symptoms persist, albeit with less severity than in the past.
- Undifferentiated – The individual's symptoms do not fit into the other categories.

PSYCHOTIC COMORBIDITIES

Disorganization of thought presents in forms outside of the discrete categories of schizophrenia and delusional disorder. Thought distortions may occur as a shared disorder, as well as a component of mood disorders. Thought disruptions can also be induced by medications and illicit substances.

Folie à Deux/Shared Psychotic Disorder

This condition, which received its name from the French for "silliness of 2," refers to a thought disruption shared by 2 or more people. One person has a delusion; a second person who interacts with the delusional person comes to accept the fixed, false belief and to share it.

Major Depressive Disorder with Psychotic Features

During a major depressive episode, the person's mood may drop so dramatically that thoughts become disorganized. The individual may develop auditory hallucinations or delusions of persecution. Such individuals may become so disorganized that they must be prescribed an antipsychotic medication as well as an antidepressant to facilitate a return from a deep depression that has caused psychotic thinking and behaviors.

Manic Psychosis

The manic episode of bipolar disorder often leads to disorganization in thought processes. The individual may suffer from hallucinations, most commonly auditory, and delusions, typically grandiose or paranoid in nature.

Schizoaffective Disorder

In this disease state, the individual suffers from comorbid mood and thought disorders, with the disturbances in mood and thought alternating and sometimes overlapping. Although not diagnostically pure, it could be said that these individuals suffer from schizophrenia plus either major depressive disorder or bipolar disorder. To be more technical, to meet the criteria for schizoaffective disorder, the individual must experience either hallucinations or delusions for a 2-week period with no major mood symptoms of either depression or mania.

Substance-Induced Psychotic Disorders

This condition occurs during substance intoxication or withdrawal, or within 1 month of either occurrence. Alcohol, hallucinogens, and psychostimulants are the substances typically suspected of causing this condition, although other substances may be potential culprits. The symptoms include delusions, disorganized and strange thoughts and thought processes, or hallucinations in conjunction with a history of substance abuse.

TREATING PSYCHOTIC DISORDERS

Note: Before initiating any therapy, the clinician should obtain informed consent from the patient, parent, or guardian (see Appendix 1).

Current medical belief is that psychosis is a phenomenon of hyper-dopaminergia (increase in dopamine neurotransmission, typically believed to be increased in the mesolimbic pathway). When the postsynaptic dopamine receptors are blocked, the individual's thinking reorganizes and notable lessening or a complete cessation of the delusions and hallucinations occurs. While 33% of individuals are treatment-resistant, 67% of individuals with psychosis will respond successfully to medication.

The concept of affinity, meaning the attraction of medication for the receptor site, helped shape and guide the development of newer antipsychotic medications. As research progressed, it was found that the greater the affinity for the D_2 receptor sites on the postsynaptic neurons, the greater the benefit and the lower the dose of medication needed. The concept of low-potency and high-potency antipsychotic medications is based on the medication's affinity for the postsynaptic receptor sites. The foundation for the current dopamine hypothesis of psychosis is based on (1) the concept of potency with regard to affinity for the D_2 receptor site on the postsynaptic neuron; and (2) the finding that amphetamines can produce a psychotic episode because of their ability to increase the amount of synaptic/postsynaptic dopamine (hyper-dopaminergia).

In today's medicine cabinet, there are 2 types of antipsychotic medications, typical antipsychotics and atypical antipsychotics.

Typical Antipsychotic Medications

The typical antipsychotic medications are traditional older-line medications. Thorazine (chlorpromazine) was the first antipsychotic medication, introduced in 1952 by Jean Delay and Paul Deniker, and is still prescribed today. Haldol (haloperidol) was introduced in the 1960s by the Belgian scientist Paul Janssen, who also developed Orap (pimozide) and, more recently, the atypical antipsychotic medication Risperdal (risperidone). As haloperidol has a higher affinity for the D_2 receptor site, it is dosed at a lower level than chlorpromazine, which has a much lower affinity.

Side Effects of the Typical Antipsychotic Medications. Generally, the side effects from the typical antipsychotic medications fall within 3 categories (Table 1).

Table 1. Side Effect Potential Based on Medication Potency of the Typical Antipsychotic Medications

Potency	Sedation	Anticholinergic	Extrapyramidal
Low potency	High	High	Low
High potency	Low	Low	High

- **Anticholinergic Side Effects.** Potential anticholinergic side effects include blurry vision, constipation, dry mouth, sedation, urinary retention, and weight gain.
- **Neuroleptic Malignant Syndrome.** The most frightening of all of the risks or side effects of the dopamine-blocking medications is neuroleptic malignant syndrome. This is a life-threatening side effect that can occur anytime during the course of the treatment. Its classic symptoms include:
  - Agitation
  - Akinesia (decreased movement)
  - Confusion
  - Elevated blood pressure (hypertension)

- Elevated body temperature (hyperpyrexia)
- Increased perspiring (hyperhidrosis)
- Muscle rigidity (dystonia)
- Mutism
- Rapid heart rate (tachycardia)

If any of these symptoms appear, the individual must be quickly taken to the nearest emergency department for immediate evaluation. One in 5 individuals who develop neuroleptic malignant syndrome will die. Intervention includes:
- Discontinuing the use of the antipsychotic medication
- Initiating intravenous hydration
- Possibly using a dopamine agonist such as Dantrium (dantrolene), Parlodel (bromocriptine), or Symmetrel (amantadine)
- Ordering serial creatinine phosphokinase (CPK) tests and monitoring closely as the serum levels will elevate dramatically as the condition worsens, and decline as the condition improves

- **Extrapyramidal Side Effects.** The dopamine-blocking antipsychotic medications have the potential to disturb the individual's motor function, producing any of 4 types of extrapyramidal side effects (Box 2):
1. Acute dystonic reaction results in prolonged muscle contractions or spasms that typically affect the muscles of the neck. This can also affect the posterior oropharyngeal muscles, compromising breathing and swallowing.
2. Akathisia manifests as an uncontrolled inner sense of restlessness of body or thoughts.
3. Parkinson-like side effects result in motor tremor, motor slowing, muscle rigidity, and/or loss of facial animation.
4. Tardive dyskinesia is a disturbance of motor/muscle movement often manifesting as tongue darting, facial grimacing, jaw jutting, and/or lip smacking. It typically appears late in an individual's medication therapy.

An acute dystonic reaction usually occurs within the first 5 days after initiating the medication. If this reaction occurs, often a dose of 25 to 50 mg of over-the-counter Benadryl (diphenhydramine) will bring resolution of the symptom(s). Individuals experiencing an oculogyric crisis with their eyes rolling upward or a posterior oropharyngeal spasm with a closing of the back of their throat should receive an intramuscular injection of diphenhydramine or Cogentin (benztropine) to bring a rapid resolution of these side effects. If

Box 2. Age and Gender Are Factors in Side Effects

- Elderly women are at greatest risk for antipsychotic medication–induced parkinsonism.
- Men under the age of 30 years are at greatest risk for acute dystonic reaction.
- Middle-aged women are at increased risk for akathisia.

a side effect occurs, the clinician should reconsider the medication used in treating the individual.

Akathisia and parkinson-like symptoms typically occur within the first 2 to 2 ½ months after medication is begun. These side effects are typically treated by any 1 of the following steps:

- Reducing the dose of the antipsychotic medication
- Adding a beta-blocker such as Inderal (propranolol) 10 to 20 mg 1 to 3 times a day
- Adding a benzodiazepine such as Ativan (lorazepam) 0.5 to 1mg 1 to 3 times a day
- Adding an anticholinergic medication such as Artane (trihexyphenidyl) 1 mg by mouth, then repeated in several hours as needed, not to exceed 15 mg in a 24-hour period; or Cogentin (benztropine) 1 to 2 mg by mouth 1 to 3 times per day for 1 to 2 weeks then reassessed for discontinuation.

Tardive dyskinesia is a late-appearing condition of involuntary muscle movements typically manifested by chewing-like motions of the mouth and jaw; choreoathetoid movements of the fingers, hands, and toes; facial grimacing; jaw jutting; lip smacking; and tongue darting. There may also be athetoid movements of the head, neck, and hips. Some individuals may have irregularities in swallowing and breathing. In very advanced cases, these disturbances may result in belching and grunting noises. The risk factors for the development of tardive dyskinesia as a side effect of using an antipsychotic medication are:

- Being female
- Being older
- Having a concomitant cognitive disorder
- Having a concomitant mood disorder with the thought disorder

Being vigilant for tardive dyskinesia at its earliest onset is the key to minimizing and reversing the condition. Testing for cogwheeling rigidity in the biceps tendon of the arms can identify early onset of the condition. When discovered early in its course, discontinuing the medication may result in cessation. Sometimes merely lowering the dose is all that is necessary. If the individual has just begun taking the antipsychotic medication at the initial dosage when tardive dyskinesia occurs, then the medication should be discontinued. If the individual is taking a higher dose, it should be tapered downward and the effects assessed. After long-term use, sometimes lowering the dose will exacerbate the symptoms of tardive dyskinesia. It is thought that the potential for this condition, as well as the other extrapyramidal side effects, is lessened by using one of the atypical antipsychotic medications (see below).

Atypical Antipsychotic Medications

The original typical antipsychotic medications, while having provided benefits to individuals since first coming onto the medical scene in 1952, are not without their risks and side effects as noted. While the symptoms of schizophrenia are thought to be caused by an increase in dopamine, the blockade of dopamine receptors by the treating medications in the pursuit of treating schizophrenia, has the potential to create side effects. There are 4 dopamine pathways:

- Mesocortical pathway – This pathway is involved in motivation and emotional response. This pathway is thought to be associated with the negative symptoms of schizophrenia. Its disruption by schizophrenia creates alogia, avolition, and flat affect.
- Mesolimbic pathway – This pathway is associated with desire and reward. Its disruption is thought to be responsible for the positive symptoms of schizophrenia.
- Nigrostriatal pathway – This pathway is part of the system known as the basal ganglia motor loop. While thought to be undisturbed by the disease of schizophrenia, dopamine blockade by medication has the potential to create the motor movement side effects of parkinsonian-like tremor; the long-term motor movement dysfunction of tardive dyskinesia; the aggravating, frightening, and sometimes life-threatening symptoms of

acute dystonia; the frustrating symptoms of akathisia; and the potentially lethal neuroleptic malignant syndrome.

- Tuberoinfundibular pathway – This pathway regulates the secretion of prolactin from the anterior pituitary gland. While thought to be undisturbed by the disease of schizophrenia, dopamine blockade by medication has the potential to cause disturbances in sexual functioning, gynecomastia in men, and galactorrhea in women.

As a result, the search has continued for medications with fewer side effects. Since the 1950s and the introduction of chlorpromazine, each decade has seen the introduction of new antipsychotic medications, both typical and atypical types:

- Prolixin (fluphenazine), Stelazine (trifluoperazine), Mellaril (thioridazine), and Trilafon (perphenazine) presented in the 1960s.
- Moban (molindone) presented in the 1970s with the promise of less weight gain.
- Loxitane (loxapine), developed in the 1980s, proved to have dual beneficial actions. It improved thought disturbances as an antipsychotic and also improved mood as an antidepressant.
- In 1990, the era of the atypical antipsychotic medication began with approval by the US Food and Drug Administration (FDA) of Clozaril (clozapine), developed by Novartis. This was followed quickly by Janssen's Risperdal (risperidone, approved in 1993), Lilly's Zyprexa (olanzapine, 1996), and AstraZeneca's Seroquel (quetiapine, 1997).
- Pfizer introduced Geodon (ziprasidone) in 2001 and Bristol-Myers Squibb partnered with Otsuka to introduce Abilify (aripiprazole, a partial dopamine agonist) in 2002.

The atypical antipsychotic medications are currently FDA approved for treating thought disorders and bipolar disorder. Risperidone has also been approved to treat irritability in children and adolescents with autism. These medications are currently prescribed off-label for treating anxiety and aggressive behavior.

The atypical antipsychotics were introduced to provide greater benefit with fewer side effects. While greater benefit may have been achieved, and while many of the atypical antipsychotic medications may cause fewer side effects, they are not without risks. Clozapine has been effective for many nonresponders to the typical antipsychotic medications, yet approximately 1% of individuals taking clozapine are at risk of developing agranulocytosis, a potentially lethal blood disorder.

The newer medications are more selective in targeting the dopamine receptors. Because the nigrostriatal system is responsible for movement disturbances, the atypical antipsychotic medications seek to more specifically target the meso-limbic system. While the typical antipsychotic medications are thought to take more of a shotgun approach to dopamine receptor sites D_1 through D_5, the atypical antipsychotics seek to selectively block the postsynaptic dopamine receptors D_1, D_2, and D_4. While the atypical antipsychotic medications are thought to have less potential for extrapyramidal side effects, neuroleptic malignant syndrome and tardive dyskinesia, new questions arise as to their impact on cardiac function, cholesterol levels, glucose metabolism, and triglyceride levels.

Individuals taking risperidone should be monitored for signs of akathisia. Olanzapine can produce significant weight gain in individuals. While quetiapine supposedly has less weight gain potential than risperidone or olanzapine, individuals taking quetiapine must be monitored for cardiac function, specifically prolongation of the QT_c. Ziprasidone also has less weight gain potential, as well as less potential for extrapyramidal side effects; however, it may bring about prolongation of the QT_c (Box 3).

Box 3. The QT_c

The QT_c is the rate-corrected QT interval, representing the time required for depolarization and repolarization of the cardiac tissue. The risk of cardiac dysrhythmias increases when the QT interval is prolonged beyond 450 msec. The 2 most often occurring dysrhythmias are ventricular fibrillation and *torsades de pointes* ("twisting of the points"). It is possible that these 2 cardiac dysrhythmias are responsible for sudden death syndrome.

Researchers believe the prolongation of the QT interval is related to the antagonism of 1 or more ion channels in the cardiac cells. For example, haloperidol antagonizes the potassium channels, pimozide the calcium channels, and chlorpromazine the sodium channels.

Weight Gain from Atypical Antipsychotic Medications. There are several off-label approaches to blocking the weight gain from atypical antipsychotic medications.

- **H$_2$ Blockers**. Recent studies have shown the use of a histamine$_2$ blocker such as Axid (nizatidine) and Tagamet (cimetidine) to be beneficial in blocking the weight gain caused by use of the atypical antipsychotic medications. The greatest benefit from nizatidine was shown to occur at 300 mg daily, while cimetidine proved most beneficial at 150 mg twice a day. While the mechanism of action for offsetting weight gain is not well understood, one hypothesis presented is that the histamine$_2$ blocker may calm gastrointestinal upset that the individuals intuitively self-medicate by eating more food.

- **Topamax (topiramate)**. This antiseizure medication inhibits weight gain and has become popular to treat individuals taking atypical antipsychotic medications. It has also been noted clinically to help stabilize mood. Individuals should be monitored for cognitive impact when taking topiramate. While individuals may report cognitive dulling at lower dosing ranges, this cognitive impact typically occurs at doses of 200 mg per day. Individuals should be advised to report any eye pain, as this may be a symptom of the rare side effect of medication-induced glaucoma-like phenomenon. Individuals should report any paradoxical irritability. There have also been reports of kidney stones (nephrolithiasis) in individuals using topiramate, so individuals should drink 8 glasses of water a day and report any flank pain.

  Topiramate is started at 25 mg by mouth in the evening and then increased to twice a day dosing after 3 days. Some individuals may need to have their dosing regimen increased to 50 mg twice a day to achieve weight control.

- **Wellbutrin (bupropion)**. Researchers at Duke University have found that individuals lost weight when using bupropion. The medication is also noted to have minimal potential for mood cycling in individuals who might have bipolar disorder. Bupropion improves focus and concentration, increases energy, and has been noted to reverse sexual dysfunction caused by use of serotonin selective reuptake inhibitor medications.

- **Zonegran (zonisamide)**. FDA approved as adjunctive therapy for adult partial seizures, this antiseizure medication has been shown to effect weight loss. Zonisamide is usually dosed at 25 mg 1 to 2 times a day to achieve this benefit.

Versatility of the Atypical Antipsychotic Medications. The atypical antipsychotics were originally developed to provide relief from psychosis by treating both positive and negative symptoms. Generally, these medications offer a better safety profile for individuals, with more focused receptor site targeting, than typical antipsychotic medications. These medications are also FDA approved for treating the mood lability of bipolar disorder. In addition, clinicians prescribe the atypical antipsychotic medications off-label for treating:

- Anxiety in adults
- Aggression in elderly residents of nursing facilities; these individuals' cardiac health should be closely monitored, however, as concerns have arisen over the increase in cardiac misadventures in elderly individuals taking the atypical antipsychotics
- Behavioral acting out in children with attention-deficit/hyperactivity disorder and adolescents with oppositional defiant disorder and conduct disorder (see Chapter 8)
- Insomnia for individuals who do not respond to other sleep-facilitating medications

Reasons for Switching from a Typical Antipsychotic to an Atypical Antipsychotic Medication. Although typical antipsychotic medications have a long history of providing benefit and are still beneficial to many individuals, clinicians may find the atypical medications have numerous advantages for their psychotic individuals:

- Atypical antipsychotic medications improve both negative and positive symptoms in psychotic disorders.
- Atypical antipsychotic medications, being both dopaminergic and serotonergic in action, treat both the thought disorder and comorbid mood disorder.
- Atypical antipsychotic medications are less anticholinergic than their typical counterparts. This spares individuals from the confusion and cognitive dulling often accompanying the anticholinergic component.
- Atypical antipsychotic medications are thought to provide longer benefit with less potential for disease recurrence than the typical antipsychotic medications. As the atypical medications have fewer side effects, individual adherence to the medication regimen is better, decreasing the likelihood of disease recurrence.

Monitoring Risks and Side Effects of All Antipsychotic Medications

Individual safety is paramount. Individuals who are acutely psychotic should be treated in the hospital. The key to safely prescribing antipsychotic medications, whether typical or atypical, is to be aware of their potential risks and side effects. As long as an individual is taking an antipsychotic medication, the clinician should carry out and chart the results for the following 6-point test every time the individual is seen.

1. Observe the individual walking in front of you to assess for any gait disturbance(s) or truncal carriage disturbance(s). Watch for natural arm swing or lack thereof. This information can easily be obtained as the individual and clinician are walking from the waiting room to the office just prior to beginning the formal session.

2. Have the individual extend his or her arms to the front with fingers separated and extended. Observe for any tremor of the arms, hands, or fingers.

3. Moving from the larger picture to smaller movements, have the individual perform the following test, first with one hand and then the other: Ask the individual to touch the tips of his or her fingers to the tip of the thumb of that hand, going from index finger, to middle finger, to ring finger, to little finger, and then back again from little finger to index finger. Then have the individual do this with the other hand. Observe for 2 phenomena:
   a. Monitor the hand being tested to observe for smoothness and ease of dexterity.
   b. Monitor the other hand, which should be quiescent, and observe for any mirroring of motion. This may be a soft neurologic sign of some other underlying learning disability or disturbance.

4. Test for dysdiadochokinesia by asking the individual to place his or her hands together palm to palm to test rapid alternating motion. The test begins by touching the palm of the right hand to the palm of the left hand. Then the individual lifts and turns the right hand so that the back of it is now in the left palm; the individual then rapidly returns to the palm-to-palm position. The individual does this movement rapidly 4 or 5 times, and then repeats the process by changing the hand that is doing the palm-to-palm, back-to-palm, palm-to-palm maneuver. Again, monitor for dexterity and smoothness of motion.

5. Ask permission to take the individual's arms through passive range of motion in pump-handle fashion. Place your index finger or thumb into the antecubital fossa and feel for any cogwheeling rigidity/ratcheting of the biceps tendon as you move the individual's forearm, with palm upward, toward the bicep. Move the arm passively up and down several times in pump-handle fashion. This may provide the earliest sign of onset of tardive dyskinesia. When the signs are diagnosed at this point, medication dose can be lowered, discontinued, or changed, and the condition can be avoided.

6. Have the individual protrude his or her tongue and observe for tremor and/ or fasciculations.

This 6-point test is an analogue to the AIMS (abnormal involuntary movement scale) test. If any disturbances are present, the clinician should suspect the onset of tardive dyskinesia. In such a case, if the individual is receiving benefit from the medication, the clinician can lower the dose. If this either does not relieve the symptoms or leads to loss of benefit, or both, then the medication will need to be changed and the individual monitored closely.

Metabolic Syndrome

While the underlying cause of the cluster of metabolic disturbances termed *metabolic syndrome* is unknown, and while the diagnostic criteria are not universally standardized, the condition known as metabolic syndrome has been seen in some individuals taking atypical antipsychotic medications. The relationship between atypical antipsychotics and metabolic syndrome is still not well defined. At the time of the publication of this book (2009), it is thought important to monitor individuals taking atypical antipsychotics for the symptoms of metabolic syndrome, because of the potential for the individual to develop diabetes mellitus and cardiovascular disease. The factors to monitor are blood pressure, fasting plasma glucose, high-density lipoprotein cholesterol, triglycerides, and waist circumference. The levels indicative of metabolic syndrome are:

- Blood pressure >140/90 mm Hg (per the World Health Organization)
- Fasting plasma glucose >110 mg/dL
- High-density lipoprotein cholesterol <50 mg/dL in women, <40 mg/dL in men
- Triglycerides >150 mg/dL
- Waist circumference >35 inches in women, >40 inches in men

The individual should have baseline measurements of these 5 factors taken before starting an atypical antipsychotic medication and then be evaluated at regular intervals, especially if the individual begins to gain weight. The diagnosis of metabolic syndrome is made when 3 of the above 5 indicators reach the levels noted above. If any of the above levels are reached after an individual starts taking an antipsychotic medication, changing the medication should be strongly considered.

When a medication must be changed for any reason, it should be done in a way that does not leave the individual uncovered for the original symptoms that required the medication. The clinician must consider, for example, that tardive dyskinesia might be the lesser of 2 evils, compared with the individual's psychotic disorder. This is an issue that needs to be discussed with the individual in the beginning of and throughout treatment (see Appendix 1).

CHAPTER FOUR

Substance Disorders

There are substantial differences between illicit substances and prescription medications. Illicit substances are made in unregulated laboratory conditions and manufactured to no given set of standards with the expressed intention of illegal street distribution. A clinician writes for prescription medications, which are manufactured in a safe setting to US Food and Drug Administration (FDA) standards and requirements. In order of preference, the substances most commonly abused are:

- Alcohol
- Cigarettes and other tobacco products (nicotine)
- Marijuana (cannabis sativa); the Federal government lists marijuana as an illicit substance, according to the Harrison Act of 1914. It has been "medicalized" in 11 states, as of March 2005
- Prescription medications and illicit methamphetamine; as of 2005, illicit methamphetamine ("meth") use surpassed the illicit use of cocaine in popularity (Table 1)

Table 1. Common Substances/Medications of Abuse

Category	Examples
Alcohol	Liquor, beer, cough formulations
Anxiolytics (anti-anxiety medications)	Benzodiazepines
Caffeine	Coffee, cola drinks, chocolate
Cannabinoids	Marijuana
Hallucinogens	LSD, mushrooms, peyote
Inhalants	Gasoline, paints, propellants
Nicotine	Cigarettes, cigars, chewing tobacco, snuff
Opiates (pain medications)	Codeine, heroin, hydromorphone, meperidine
Psychostimulants	Amphetamines, cocaine, methamphetamine, methylphenidate
Sedatives/Hypnotics	Barbiturates and nonbarbiturates

THREE EFFECTS IMPLICATED IN ADDICTION

Unfortunately, prescription medications may be diverted from legal use to illegal street use (Box 1). Regardless of where manufactured, to what specifications, and where sold, both illicit substances and prescription medications can have the potential to create tolerance, dependence, and withdrawal. These 3 factors can affect compliance by individuals taking prescription medications. As noted previously, for both prescription medications and illicit substances, these 3 factors can lead to addiction (Box 2).

Box 1. Prescription Medication Abuse

Street diversion, which may be an issue with some medications, is the movement of a medication from its appropriate, prescribed, medical use, to its sale on the street for illicit purposes. Medications that can be crushed and introduced into the body intranasally have the greatest potential for street diversion for abuse, especially if they offer the user a "buzz."

An example of prescription medications being diverted to street use includes the psychostimulant medications used to treat attention-deficit/hyperactivity disorder (ADHD) and excessive daytime sleepiness (EDS). Psychiatric medications used to treat ADHD and EDS, both on label and off-label, with minimal potential for street diversion include:

- **Concerta (methylphenidate)** – A psychostimulant, this medication comes in a capsule form with an internal paste that cannot be crushed and snorted. Destruction of the capsule actually destroys the medication delivery system. This medication is FDA approved for treating ADHD in children, adolescents, and adults.
- **Imipramine** –When used to treat ADHD, this tricyclic antidepressant medication does not provide a "dopamine rush."
- **Provigil (modafinil)** – This is not a traditional psychostimulant. This medication is FDA approved for treating the excessive daytime sleepiness resulting from Obstructive Sleep Apnea/Hypopnea Syndrome

Box 1 Continued

The Goldman Guide to Psychiatry

(OSA/HS), Narcolepsy, and Shift Work Sleep Disorder (SWSD). It focuses on the sleep-wake center in the hypothalamus, has minimal activity in the nucleus accumbens and the ventral tegmental area, and does not provide a dopamine rush.

- **Strattera (atomoxetine)** – This non-psychostimulant FDA approved for treating ADHD in children, adolescents, and adults, focuses on blocking the reuptake of norepinephrine and does not provide a dopamine rush.
- **Vyvanse (lisdexamfetamine)** – This psychostimulant is a prodrug, meaning it is inactive until activated in the intestinal tract. Lysine is added to the active dexamphetamine. In the intestinal tract, the lysine is cleaved, leaving the active dexamphetamine component to provide the benefit in treating ADHD. Being a prodrug, it offers a safer abuse profile than a traditional amphetamine, as the contents cannot be taken via intranasal or intravenous route to achieve a "high."
- **Wellbutrin (bupropion)** – This antidepressant is used off-label for treating ADHD. It provides gentler presynaptic reuptake transport pump blockade for dopamine and does not give a dopamine rush. It also provides moderate presynaptic reuptake transport pump inhibition for norepinephrine.

The most often diverted prescription medications include the amphetamine psychostimulants, the benzodiazepines, the myriad of pain medications, and muscle relaxant medications.

Box 2. The Devastating Impact of Substance Abuse

Substance abuse is a major precipitating factor in suicide. Fifteen percent of individuals who abuse alcohol will successfully commit suicide in their foreshortened lifetime. Persons who abuse substances are 20 times more likely to commit suicide than are non–substance abusers.

Tolerance occurs as an individual no longer receives the desired effect from the same amount of medication or substance (Box 3). This results in the individual requiring more of the substance/medicine at a given time or taking the same amount more frequently. Clinicians are advised to monitor individuals for tolerance to the benzodiazepines, eg, Ativan (lorazepam), Klonopin (clonazepam), Valium (diazepam), and Xanax (alprazolam). Tolerance to pain medications is also a concern, eg, Davocet (acetaminophen/propoxyphene), OxyContin (oxycodone), Percocet (acetaminophen/oxycodone), Percodan (aspirin/oxycodone), Ultram (tramadol), and Vicodin (acetaminophen/hydrocodone).

Box 3. A Case of Tolerance

As an hypothetical case, Mr. Nervus is taking alprazolam 0.25 mg by mouth twice a day for anxiety. After 3 weeks, he is seen in a follow-up appointment and relates that his prescription has already run out. He may report he needs to take the medication 3 times a day now instead of twice a day or that he needs to take 2 of the tablets twice a day now instead of 1 tablet twice a day. This is an example of tolerance. The benefit derived from the prescribed dose of medication is no longer effective indicating tolerance is occurring. In order to achieve the desired benefit, the individual needs to increase the amount of the medication taken by increasing either the dose or the frequency of the medication or both.

When an individual stops taking a medication as prescribed and experiences serious discomfort, the clinician must consider the possibility of dependence. Of course, the discomfort can signal a resumption of the symptoms the medication was originally prescribed to treat, which represents a relapse, not withdrawal. The discomfort may also represent withdrawal symptoms.

When the individual is dependent on the medication, the body reacts negatively to its absence, leaving the system in withdrawal. With tricyclic antidepressants and benzodiazepines, the potential exists for a withdrawal seizure if an individual abruptly discontinues the medication. Anti-seizure medications are used regularly to provide mood stabilization. If an anti-seizure medication is abruptly discontinued, the individual is at risk for a withdrawal seizure, regardless of whether the individual has any history of seizures. Tapering the medication to discontinuation is the appropriate treatment approach to avoid the possibility of the withdrawal seizure.

Defining Abuse Versus Dependence

The diagnosis of dependence requires the presence of both tolerance and withdrawal symptoms. Abuse, on the other hand, is the diagnosis when the individual experiences 1 or more of the following:

- Use of the substance impairs the person's ability to perform important daily life activities at work, home, or school.
- Use of the substance occurs in places and situations that are inadvisable and put the individual or others at risk for their safety (eg, use while driving a car).
- Use of the substance results in legal consequences (eg. DUI).
- Use of the substance persists even though it is causing impairment in the person's life either in daily life functioning or in relationships at home, school, or work.

ALCOHOL ABUSE: DIAGNOSIS AND TREATMENT

Diagnosing Alcohol Abuse

The acronym **CAGE**, as incorporated into the following 4 questions, is used as a means to diagnose alcohol abuse. A positive answer to any 2 of the 4 questions indicates an alcohol abuse problem.

- **C** – Have you ever tried to **C**ut down on your use of alcohol?
- **A** – Have you ever been **A**nnoyed by people commenting about your alcohol use?
- **G** – Have you ever felt **G**uilty or worried about your use of alcohol?
- **E** – Have you ever had an **E**ye-opener drink in the morning?

Visual observation, a physical examination, and laboratory tests reveal important information to further enable a diagnosis of alcohol abuse. To diagnose the condition in its early stage, the clinician should:

1. Look for acne rosacea, commonly seen in progressing alcoholism.
2. Ask about an increase in incidence of upper respiratory tract infections.

3. Ask about the individual's involvement in legal proceedings for driving under the influence of alcohol or other intoxicating substances.
4. Ask if the individual has been involved recently in minor traffic accidents.
5. Ask if the individual is experiencing periods of blackout episodes, which are often described as "lost time."
6. Assess for reddening of the palms (palmar erythema), which results from increasing levels of circulating estrogen secondary to excessive alcohol intake.
7. Look at the individual's fingers to assess for cigarette burns.
8. Look for and ask about unexplained bruising.
9. Palpate for painless enlargement of the liver due to fatty infiltrates, the earliest form of liver disease due to alcohol.

As alcoholism advances, clinicians should conduct a physical examination for the following:
1. Cirrhosis of the liver, which occurs in 10% of alcoholics
2. Dupuytren's contractures
3. Gynecomastia
4. Jaundice or ascites
5. Testicular atrophy

Two laboratory values are key indicators of alcoholism. An elevated gamma-glutamyltranspeptidase (GGT) level occurs in 75% of alcohol abusers as an early sign of abuse. The mean corpuscular volume (MCV) is elevated in approximately 95% of alcohol abusers. Overall, 90% of alcohol abusers will demonstrate an elevation in both the GGT and MCV values.

Serious Effects of Long-Term Alcohol Abuse

Wernicke's encephalopathy is an acute and reversible condition caused by a thiamine (vitamin B1) deficiency. In individuals who significantly abuse alcohol, the deficiency can occur because of poor nutrition caused by the consumption of alcohol instead of food. To diagnose this condition, the clinician should look for ataxia, confusion, and horizontal nystagmus. The condition is treated with 100 mg of intramuscular thiamine.

Wernicke-Korsakoff syndrome is Wernicke's encephalopathy taken to the next level of severity. The individual suffers from a chronic impairment in memory and cognitive function. The condition is reversible in one-third of individuals. In two-thirds of those suffering from this syndrome, it is an irreversible condition. The lack of adequate nutrition brought on by excessive alcohol consumption adversely impacts cognitive function. The hallmark of this condition is confabulation demonstrated when these individuals respond to questions by giving answers that are created out of thin air.

Treating Alcohol Abuse

Note: Before initiating any therapy, the clinician should obtain informed consent from the individual, parent, or guardian (see Appendix1).

Uncomplicated withdrawal from alcohol is similar to caffeine withdrawal, in that the individual experiences discomfort once the substance is no longer available. The individual may experience mild tremors approximately 12 to 18 hours after the last ingestion of alcohol, which peak after 1 or 2 days. The individual returns to some level of homeostasis within 5 to 7 days.

Complicated withdrawal occurs if the individual experiences seizures. In older literature and street parlance, alcohol withdrawal seizures were called rum fits. Complicated withdrawal usually occurs within 7 to 36 hours after cessation of alcohol. If the individual has been drinking large amounts for a long period of time, he or she may experience withdrawal hallucinations that begin approximately 2 days after cessation of alcohol and last approximately 7 days.

The extreme form of alcohol withdrawal is delirium tremens, which usually occurs following complicated withdrawal seizures. The individual will manifest autonomic dysregulation, confusion, and tremors. Delirium tremens begins approximately 2 to 3 days after the last drink, peaks in 4 to 5 days, and may last for several weeks. In its most severe form, delirium tremens can be fatal.

To avoid all of these symptoms, individuals can be placed on a withdrawal protocol. Typically, this involves prescribing Librium (chlordiazepoxide) at 25 to

Table 2. Alcohol Withdrawal Types and Symptoms

TYPES OF WITHDRAWAL	SYMPTOMS	ONSET	PEAK	RESOLUTION
Uncomplicated	Discomfort	12-18 hours	1-2 days	5-7 days
Complicated	Seizures (rum fits)	7-36 hours	2-7 days	7 days
Extreme	Delirium tremens	2-3 days	4-5 days	2 weeks

50 mg 4 times a day for 1 day, and then tapering over the following 4 to 5 days. If the individual suffers from severe liver injury due to years of alcohol insult, Ativan (lorazepam) or Serax (oxazepam) may be used as the benzodiazepine protocol of choice. These 2 benzodiazepines have minimal metabolite trace and clear through the kidneys (renal clearance). Individuals who experience hallucinations can also receive small doses of an antipsychotic medication.

Treatment to Avoid Relapse. Once the individual is through the withdrawal period, it is important to help the individual avoid returning to the use of alcohol. Participation in support groups such as Alcoholics Anonymous is critical. Clinicians can also prescribe any of the following FDA approved medications to assist in maintaining abstinence in the recovering alcoholic:

- **Antabuse (disulfiram)**. Disulfiram serves as an inhibitor of acetaldehyde dehydrogenase (AAD), an enzyme that breaks down alcohol. When AAD is inhibited, acetaldehyde builds up, inducing extremely discomforting symptoms such as drop in blood pressure, heart palpitations, nausea, and vomiting. The typical dose is 250 mg per day. If individuals take this medication at the same time as they ingest alcohol, they may experience a violent illness response.
- **Campral (acamprosate)**. Acamprosate enhances the balance in the brain between the excitatory neurotransmitter glutamate and the inhibitory neurotransmitter gamma-amino butyric acid. It is dosed as 666 mg by mouth 3 times per day as two 333-mg tablets per dosing period. This medication can be taken even if the individual relapses into use of alcohol. Its concurrent use during a relapse may lessen the severity and length of the relapse and speed the individual's return to recovering status.
- **ReVia (naltrexone)**. Naltrexone is a mu opioid antagonist that reduces the psychologically reinforcing pleasurable effects of alcohol, thereby decreasing the individual's desire for alcohol. The recommended daily dose is 50 mg by mouth each day.
- **Vivitrol (injectible sustained-release naltrexone)**. This injectible form of naltrexone was FDA approved in 2006. It is given intramuscularly once a month with the dose being 380 mg per injection.

NICOTINE ABUSE

After alcohol abuse, nicotine is the most commonly abused substance. Nicotine is a highly addictive substance commonly found in tobacco products. Its most common introduction is via cigarettes. An estimated 1 in 4 American adults smoke cigarettes. Individuals with schizophrenia have the highest rate of cigarette use in the population, with approximately 90% of those diagnosed with schizophrenia smoking cigarettes. As nicotine stimulates the release of dopamine in the brain, it is thought that schizophrenic individuals intuitively smoke cigarettes to offset side effects caused by their dopamine-blocking anti-psychotic medications.

Nicotine is highly addictive and has rapid onset of withdrawal symptoms, as quickly as 1 hour after the last cigarette has been smoked. Nicotine withdraw-al peaks within 24 hours of the last use of cigarettes. The withdrawal from nicotine is long-lived, lasting from weeks to months. Nicotine withdrawal is highlighted by craving for another cigarette, mood lability and irritability, feel-ings of anxiousness, and feelings of restlessness. Because of the decrease in dopamine release, individuals discontinuing cigarette use commonly experi-ence weight gain and decrease in mood.

Treatment Approaches to Facilitate Cigarette Discontinuation

A number of medications, both prescription and over-the-counter, are currently available to help smokers "break the habit."

- **Chantix (varenicline)**. This prescription medication has a dual mechanism of action. It blocks the nicotine receptor sites and provides mild release of dopamine, to help take the place of nicotine's impact in the brain. Clinicians must monitor this medication for changes in mood and/or suicidal ideations.
- **Nicotine-Tapering Medications**. Both transdermal nicotine patches and nicotine-containing gum are used to replace the nicotine from the discon-tinued cigarettes. The amount of nicotine received is tapered slowly to complete discontinuation.
- **Zyban (bupropion hydrochloride)**. This prescription medication is the same formulation as Wellbutrin (bupropion hydrochloride), the antidepres-sant. It blocks the presynaptic reuptake transport pump for dopamine, thus providing greater availability of dopamine in the brain. The role played by this medication is to simulate the release of dopamine achieved by smoking cigarettes.

Relapse rates are very high among individuals attempting to stop smoking cigarettes. Often adding the non-pharmacologic approaches of hypnosis or acupuncture to the pharmacologic treatments enhances the success rate.

CHAPTER FIVE

Suicide and Violent Behavior

THE BASICS OF SUICIDE

Suicide is the self-infliction of death, intentional rather than accidental (Box 1). In his book *Definitions of Suicide* (John Wiley & Sons, 1985), Edwin Schneidman defines suicide as

> the conscious act of self-induced annihilation, best understood as a multidimensional malaise in a needful individual who defines an issue for which the act is perceived as the best solution (p 203).

The single greatest predictor of an individual's potential for suicide is past suicide attempts. The most important question a clinician can ask an individual to assist in determining suicidal potential is "Are you having any thoughts of wanting to hurt yourself, wanting to die, or wanting to kill yourself?"

Contrary to social myth, asking an individual if he or she is having suicidal thoughts will not implant those thoughts into the individual's mind. Asking about suicidal thoughts may, however, uncover the individual's current thoughts of committing suicide.

Eight of 10 persons who eventually succeed at suicide give warnings of their intentions, with 50% saying openly that they want to die. When an individual admits to a plan of action, this is a dangerous sign. If individuals who have been threatening suicide become quiet and less agitated, this may be an ominous sign that they have made peace with their intent to die and are starting to pursue the suicidal act.

After an attempt has occurred, it is important to assess the lethality or seriousness of the attempt:

HOW it was attempted + **WHERE** it was attempted = **Potential of Lethality**

Box 1: Suicide Facts

- 30,000 individuals die from suicide each year in the United States (attempted suicides are estimated to be 8 to 10 times that number).
- Someone successfully commits suicide every 18 minutes in the United States.
- Suicide is the 2nd leading cause of death for individuals aged 15 to 24 years and the 8th most frequent cause of death in adults overall. Ranking in order of cause of death:

    1. Heart disease
    2. Cancer
    3. Cerebrovascular disease
    4. Accidents
    5. Pneumonia
    6. Diabetes mellitus
    7. Cirrhosis
    8. Suicide

- Women attempt suicide 3:1 to men; men succeed in suicide 3:1 to women.
- Married people are less likely to commit suicide than are single, divorced, or widowed persons.
- Nearly one-third of suicides occur in persons with chronic alcoholism and 90% have alcohol in their bloodstream at the time of death.
- About 5% of those who successfully commit suicide have serious physical illnesses at the time of suicide.
- The suicide rate in individuals with acquired immunodeficiency syndrome (AIDS) in the United States is 7 times that of the general population.
- 30% of those who successfully commit suicide have a history of past suicide attempts.
- 1 in 6 suicide victims leaves a note.
- Two-thirds of those who commit suicide will communicate their suicidal intentions to others.
- Psychiatric individuals remain at high risk for suicide after hospital discharge. Relapse can happen quickly.
- The risk of suicide as the cause of death is much higher among psychiatric patients than in the general population.
- The 10% to 15% rule suggests 10% to 15% of individuals with bipolar disorder, major depressive disorder, or schizophrenia will successfully commit suicide.

The Goldman Guide to Psychiatry

- **HOW** determines the potential reversibility of the attempt. Refusing to eat for a day is different from ingesting an entire bottle of pills. The type of pills taken is material to the potential lethality of the attempt. The use of a firearm adds a further dimension of potential permanency to the suicide attempt.

- **WHERE** impacts the potential for a rescuer to intervene. The potential lethality for the individual who takes a handful of pills in front of his or her mother in the kitchen is much different from the potential lethality for the individual who goes into the forest, miles from any other person, places a handgun into his or her mouth, and pulls the trigger.

As noted, asking an individual of his or her suicidal ideations will not implant the idea of self-harm; it may certainly uncover an underlying intent to die that is not readily volunteered. Questions about thoughts of self-harm are plain and direct:

- Are you having any thoughts of dying?
- Are you having any thoughts of wanting to kill yourself?
- When was the last time you had these thoughts?
- Have you ever acted on these thoughts before? If so, please describe what you did.
- Do you have a plan now? If so, what is it?
- Do you currently have the intent to act on the plan?
- Do you have the tools to implement your plan?

The purpose of these questions is to determine where the individual's suicidal ideations lie on a passive-to-active continuum. On the passive side is the individual who says if he were standing on the street corner and a bus jumped the curb and killed him, it would be okay. On the active side, the individual reports that the 3 o'clock bus comes by her street corner every afternoon. She has decided she will step off the curb in front of it tomorrow. Passive means individuals would just like to fall asleep and not wake up. Active means individuals are willing to use their energy to create a plan and implement it for their own demise.

The Suicidal Continuum
The suicidal chain of events has several levels that possess increasing detail and potential lethality:

Suicidal ideation
Suicidal ideation + Plan
Suicidal ideation + Plan + Intent
Suicidal ideation + Plan + Intent + Means
Suicidal ideation + Plan + Intent + Means + Attempt (assess the How and the Where)

The clinician can assess the individual's level on the continuum by evaluating his or her answers to the above questions in light of the following questions:

1. Does the individual have suicidal intent, i.e., the active desire to fulfill the suicidal ideation?
2. Has the individual formulated a well–thought out suicidal plan?
3. Does the individual have the actual means within his or her control to act on the plan?

If an individual is imminently suicidal and antidepressant medication(s) has not been effective, the clinician should consider electroconvulsive therapy for rapid relief of overwhelming depression and suicidal ideations with intent (see Chapter 3 and Chapter 12).

VIOLENT BEHAVIOR

In today's society, violence has become less the exception and more of a common occurrence. This is evidenced by the number of violent acts reported every day in the newspaper and on television news. Psychiatrists and other physicians and clinicians are called on regularly to make assessments of an individual's potential for violent behavior and to determine appropriate courses of treatment. When assessing individuals for their violent potential for either self-harm or harming others, clinicians should be aware of the following factors:

- The single best predictor of future violence in an individual is a past history of violent behavior.
- One of the strongest predictors of adult violence is childhood aggression.
- Alcohol is strongly associated with violent behavior and violent acts because it chemically disrupts cognition, judgment, mood, and perception.

At a physiologic level, aggressive behavior toward self (suicide) and others (homicide) is correlated with a low cerebrospinal fluid level of 5-hydroxyindoleacetic acid. While this deficiency is associated with aggressive behavior, it is thought to actually be a marker for impulsivity, rather than violence.

Behaviors commonly associated with violence include:
- Anger dysregulation
- Command auditory hallucinations
- History of prior acts of violence
- Impulsive behavior (history of attention-deficit/hyperactivity disorder)
- Paranoid ideations (psychosis)
- Personality disorder including antisocial personality disorder and borderline personality disorder
- Presence of alcohol, drug intoxication, delirium, or dementia
- Verbalized intention to harm another

Self-Injurious Behavior

Studies show that 4% of all individuals in psychiatric hospitals have cut on themselves, with a sex ratio of 3:1 women: men. This act is usually performed in private, done delicately or carefully, and explained as relieving anger or tension. Areas commonly cut are the wrists, arms, thighs, and legs. Also cut are the face, abdomen, and breasts.

Most individuals who self-inflict cuts ("cutters") deny they are seeking to die; however, most have engaged in prior suicide attempts. Cutting is commonly found among those with borderline personality disorder. Hypotheses presented for the neurobiological cause of self-injurious behaviors include:

- A decrease in serotonin levels, which is associated with impulsivity and aggressivity. Serotonin selective reuptake inhibitor medications, while not approved by the US Food and Drug Administration (FDA) for self-injurious behavior, are often the first-line treatment approach.
- Fluctuations in endogenous opioid levels. It is thought these individuals may be addicted to the high levels and elevate the levels by engaging in acts of self-injury, causing the brain to respond by releasing larger amounts of endogenous opioids. Naltrexone is prescribed for blocking the increased release of opioids.
- Dysregulation of dopaminergic activity. Atypical antipsychotic medications are used to block dopamine receptor sites.

To date there are no medications specifically FDA approved for treating self-injurious behavior. The alpha$_2$ agonists, eg, clonidine and Tenex (guanfacine), have shown success in some individuals. Mood stabilizers have also shown benefit in calming impulsivity. Antidepressants are used to improve mood and calm impulsivity.

CHAPTER SIX

Personality Disorders

Personality is the total emotional and behavioral complex of the individual. It is usually stable and predictable. Personality is the fibers woven into a fabric causing men and women to be who they are.

Personality disorders affect an individual's thinking and perception, mood responses and mood stability, interactions with others, and ability to control impulses. A disturbance in any 2 of these areas constitutes the criteria for making a diagnosis of a personality disorder. These disorders are major variants of character traits ordinarily found in most people. The traits are exaggerated, a caricature as it were; the individual becomes inflexible and maladapted, causing either functional impairment or subjective distress. Individuals with these disorders show deeply ingrained, inflexible, and maladaptive patterns in interpersonal relationships and in perceiving their environment and themselves.

Personality disorders have been divided into 3 diagnostic subset groups, designated as clusters A, B, and C.

Cluster A is comprised of the following personality disorder types:

- **Paranoid personality disorder** is defined by a long-standing suspicion and distrust of others. These individuals assign responsibility to others for all the wrongs that have befallen them and do not easily forget what they perceive to be an insult. These individuals doubt the loyalty of others and believe that half the world is out to take advantage of the other half.

- **Schizoid personality disorder** is defined by a lifelong pattern of social withdrawal. These individuals tend to be uncomfortable with human interaction and are viewed as eccentric, isolated, and lonely. These individuals are emotionally unattached, lack any close friends, and have little interest in intimacy or sexual closeness with another person.

- **Schizotypal personality disorder** is defined by exceedingly odd behavior, ideas, and presentation to others. These individuals keep to themselves and have magical thinking. They can be considered to have a small amount of paranoid personality disorder plus a dash of schizoid personality disorder. In addition, they often believe in the magical elements of the universe: extra-sensory perception, astrology, numerology, and many of the other occult and arcane disciplines. As a result, they are often victims of unethical charlatans who prey on their beliefs.

Cluster B is comprised of the following personality disorder types:

- **Borderline personality disorder** has the hallmarks of instability in relationships and self-identity, and unchecked impulsivity. These individuals figuratively stand on the border between neurosis and psychosis. They are extraordinarily unstable in affect, mood, behavior, object relations, and self-image. This results from instability in their sense of self and relationship to others, feelings of emptiness, and recurrent feelings of abandonment, causing them to be prone to recurrent suicidal acts. These individuals are also prone to self-cutting and other self-inflicted injurious behaviors (see Chapter 5). Because these individuals have a disturbed concept of boundaries, they are prone to inappropriate and intense episodes of anger and temper outbursts.

- **Antisocial personality disorder** is not synonymous with criminality. The individual is unable to respect the rights of others or to conform to social norms. These individuals tend to be warm, ingratiating, and charming—they are the confidence ("con") artists who easily win over their victims and fleece them of money, services, or emotional attachment. At times these individuals may show irritability and aggressiveness, and they usually fail to honor their financial obligations.

- **Histrionic personality disorder** is characterized by theatrical and dramatic behavior. These individuals are often described as flamboyant, outgoing, and colorful as they seek to be the center of attention. They are unable to maintain deep, long-lasting relationships; their emotions tend to be shallow and erratic. These individuals tend to be sexually seductive and read deeper meaning into relationships than what is most likely present.

- **Narcissistic personality disorder** manifests with the individual being self-centered, egocentric, and having a heightened sense of self-importance with grandiose feelings of being unique. These individuals see themselves as special, require the admiration of others, and are unable to recognize the needs of others. Individuals with narcissistic personality disorder become enraged when they are questioned or embarrassed. The narcissistic insult will cause them to cloak themselves in the aphorism "the best defense is a strong offense."

Cluster C is comprised of the following personality disorder types:

- **Dependent personality disorder** moves individuals to subordinate their needs to those of others, lack self-confidence, and feel uncomfortable being alone. These individuals are unable to make decisions without an excessive amount of advice and reassurance from others and are hesitant to express their own opinions for fear of losing the approval and support of others. If a close relationship is terminated, these individuals must immediately create a new close relationship for fear of being unable to care for themselves. They will volunteer for even the most unpleasant of tasks in the belief this will garner the support of others.

- **Obsessive-compulsive personality disorder** is characterized by emotional constriction, orderliness, perseveration, stubbornness, and indecisiveness. This is the individual who is overly devoted to work to the exclusion of leisure activities, even when income is not an issue. The hallmark is the pervasive pattern of perfectionism and inflexibility. Sufferers are so rigid and driven that they are unable to delegate responsibilities to others unless the other person performs to their rigid specifications. These individuals have difficulty discarding worn-out objects, even those that possess no sentimental value. This is the individual who is referred to in the vernacular as "being anal." This is not obsessive-compulsive disorder, which is hallmarked by the thought (the obsession) followed by the action (the compulsion) that is meant to relieve the underlying anxiety. Obsessive-compulsive personality disorder is not a discrete disease state, it is a personality disorder; therefore, it is a pervasive personality complex.

- **Passive-aggressive personality disorder** is characterized by behavior that uses passivity to express aggression, not by fluctuating from passive to aggressive behaviors. For example, a mother tells her son to clean his room. He says, "Okay, Mom, not a problem." Three hours later the room is still in disarray. The mother again tells her son, "Go clean your room." He responds, "Not a problem, Mom. I will take care of it right away." It never happens. The son displays his aggressivity by not performing the task (through passive disobedience). Note: while this diagnosis was listed in the *Diagnostic and Statistical Manual of Mental Disorders, 3rd Revised Edition*, it has been dropped from the 4th edition-TR.

- **Avoidant personality disorder** is characterized by extreme sensitivity to rejection. It is this sensitivity to rejection that leads to social withdrawal, even though these individuals desperately want to be included in social events and to be socially connected. Sufferers usually have such low self-esteem and are so afraid of being rejected or embarrassed that they avoid intimate relationships or work-related social activities.

Goldman's Mnemonic to Remember the Personality Disorders

Cluster A: If students get an "A" in a course, they pass the course. A=PaSS. The "A" comes out of the word **PaSS**, denoting cluster A, and what is left is:
- **P = Paranoid**
- **S = Schizoid**
- **S = Schizotypal**

Cluster B: On Germany's Autobahn highway, drivers are allowed to drive as fast as they want. Individuals with the personality disorders in this cluster can be thought of as "running in the fast lane" in life. If the *Auto* is dropped from Autobahn, BAHN represents the 4 disorders in this cluster:
- **B = Borderline**
- **A = Antisocial**
- **H = Histrionic**
- **N = Narcissistic**

Cluster C: For Cluster C provide the letters of the alphabet sequential numerical value, so that A=1, B=2, C=3, D=4, E=5, F=6.........Z=26. Notice that C=3. Provide the main psychiatric neurotransmitters numerical value: Norepinephrine=1, Serotonin=2, Dopamine=3. C=3 for Cluster C = 3 corresponding with the neurotransmitter Dopamine = 3, therefore, Cluster C = **DOPA**mine. For mnemonic purposes therefore Cluster C = DOPA:
- **D = Dependent**
- **O = Obsessive-Compulsive**
- **P = Passive-Aggressive**
- **A = Avoidant**

CHAPTER SEVEN

Childhood and Adolescence

UNDERLYING CAUSES OF PSYCHIATRIC DISORDERS

Psychiatric disorders can occur throughout the entire lifecycle. The underlying cause of psychiatric disorders, while not fully understood, is believed to be from 1 of 3 etiologies:

- Maturational
- Biological
  - Endogenous
  - Secondary to exogenous stressors
- Maturational and biological combined

Maturational Process

Maturational processes involve physical and psychological growth and development. The developing central nervous system forms the interconnection of the sections of the brain. That interconnected wiring allows for the synchronization of actions and thoughts within appropriate social boundaries and mores. The concept of understanding social cues, processing those cues, and reacting appropriately is related to a healthy, nurturing environment with good parental modeling, as well as the successful growth and connections of the inner brain "wiring" and the proper flow of hormones, neurotransmitters, and other neurochemicals. Psychological growth and development are discussed further in the first part of this chapter. The development of the central nervous system, its wiring, and the body's neurochemistry is the focus of the second part of this chapter.

Biological Process

Disruptions in an individual's biological development can be responsible for various disease states. As discussed below, disturbances in the connectivity of sections of the brain may be the underlying etiology of Asperger's disorder and autism. Current scientific thinking discounts the interaction between child and parents during the childhood developmental stages as the cause, viewing these 2 disease states as purely biological in etiology. On the other hand, attention-deficit hyperactivity disorder is currently viewed as a neurologic disorder that, once treated pharmacologically, will respond to appropriate psychotherapeutic and family therapy interventions. Tourette's disorder is currently viewed as a neurologic disorder appropriately treated pharmacologically, although minimizing psychosocial stressors at the same time may calm the pathognomonic tics.

The biological process of disease state can take 2 forms. The endogenous biological disruption comes from within from often-unknown causes. The reason children with autism or Asperger's disorder do not develop the appropriate and necessary internal connections to read social cues and interact verbally and socially with others is still unknown. What is known is that this occurs endogenously, neurostructurally from within. Likewise, obsessive-compulsive disorder is no longer viewed as a psychological developmental disorder that pushes the child into magical thinking. Instead it is viewed as a neurostructural and neurochemical disorder.

Some biological disruptions occur secondary to an external stressor that results in internal structural and neurochemical disturbances. Depression can be either endogenous, with no identifiable psychosocial stressor, or secondary to readily identifiable psychosocial stressors that ultimately overwhelm the individual's neurologic system, resulting in a disruption of the mechanisms for neurotransmitter production, release, and/or reuptake. Bipolar disorder and schizophrenia are considered biological in etiology. Current medical explanation points to the stress-diathesis theory that external social stressors overwhelm the individual, activating an underlying biological potential for the manifestation of these disease states.

Maturational and Biological Combined

As alluded to above, some psychiatric disease states result from a combination of disruptions in the child's psychological and biological developmental processes. Anxious school refusal is believed to be underlain by a disruption in the proper parent-child relationship combined with a biological predisposition to anxiety. Current information points to developmental issues combined with structural susceptibility in the brain that causes external psychosocial stressors to result in post-traumatic stress disorder.

UNDERSTANDING HUMAN MATURATION

An individual's progression from childhood to adolescence lays the foundation for adulthood. In this process there may be derailments along the way. This chapter starts with a review of the key concepts of Sigmund Freud, Jean Piaget, and Erik Homburg Erikson with regard to the maturational stages of the child and adolescent. With this foundation, the chapter then provides a view into the psychiatric disorders most commonly associated with childhood and adolescence, along with treatment approaches for these disorders.

The 3 Maturational Theories

Freud's Stages of Development. Sigmund Freud proposed 5 stages of development.

1. The **Oral Stage**, designated from birth to 1 year old, is termed the oral stage because the infant is focused on survival via oral intake. The infant engages in feeding, sucking from either breast or bottle. At this stage the infant is gratification-driven, deriving fulfillment from oral stimulation. Freud suggests that during the oral stage, the child seeks immediate gratification. This is also the stage of greatest dependency on others as the infant is unable to care for himself or herself.

   The id is Freud's concept of the primal energy underlying the drive for survival. During the oral stage, the new being is all id. The infant focuses on the 4 tasks of crying, eating, sleeping, and toileting. The infant is egocentric with no concept of self or other, as life is all about him or her. There is no concept of time and no understanding of past, present, or future. The infant lives in the present moment. As ego evolves concurrently with id, the maturing child comes to understand the separation of self from other and the concept of time being past, present, and future.

2. The **Anal Stage** occurs from ages 1 to 3 years, when the infant evolves into toddler. Life focus progresses from the mouth to the anus. It is in this stage that the child begins to derive more pleasure from holding feces than from feeding the mouth. Toilet training occurs in this stage. Freud postulated a battle between toddler and parent for control over "letting go." Parents demand an orderly and timely letting go and the toddler seeks to "hold on." The behavioral issues are those of cleanliness versus messiness. It is the conflict between super-rigidity, causing a rigid sense of orderliness, versus being messy and defiant.

3. The **Phallic Stage** occurs from ages 4 to 6 years. Focus shifts from the anus to the genital erogenous zone. At the same time, the child shifts his or her attentions to the opposite sex parent. This is the basis of Freud's Oedipus complex (The Oedipal conflict), wherein the son wants the mother and the

daughter wants the father. This psychosexual drama resolves with 2 components. In the Oedipal conflict, the father exerts parental power that influences the son to cease and desist from intimate desires for the mother. This results in the son becoming comfortable "repressing" these sexual impulses and the son thereafter identifies with the dad. (This may be the prototype for the concept of identification with the aggressor espoused by Freud's daughter, Anna Freud.) This process solidifies the continued progress of the evolving superego, known as the conscience. From this stage, the child moves into the latency stage wherein sexuality becomes temporarily quiescent. (The female correlate is the Electra complex wherein the daughter wants the father.)

4. The **Latency Stage** occurs from 7 to 11 years of age. Freud believed the repression of the sexual impulses that had been directed toward the opposite sex parent in the previous phallic stage became generalized to the rest of the child's life during this sexually quiescent phase. The school-aged child redirects this sexual energy to studying, learning, reading, and playing with friends. Freud believed the child to be flower-like at this point, just waiting to bloom.

5. The **Genital Stage** is the stage of blooming. Freud projected this stage from the age of 11 years onward. This stage marks the onset of adolescence and puberty, when interest in the opposite sex is re-ignited and continues as a lifelong process. Freud defined this stage as the time when the individual becomes socially connected in intimate ways.

Jean Piaget's Stages of Development. Jean Piaget's developmental stages are more functionally oriented. They do not focus on development as a sexual phenomenon; Piaget viewed development as a cognitive process.

1. The **Sensorimotor Stage** occurs from age 0 to 2 years old. Fundamental to this stage is the concept of permanence. At this stage, Piaget postulated, "If you cannot see it, it isn't there." His paradigm is that of a toy ball. If the ball rolls under the couch and the child cannot see it, then to the child it no longer exists. Jean Piaget believed that around the age of 2 years, the child comes to understand that a ball that rolls under the couch is still a ball. It still exists; it is simply under the couch. At this stage, the child comes to understand object permanence.

2. The **Preoperational Stage** occurs from ages 2 to 7 years. In this stage the child develops symbols for objects, that is, language. The child is egocentric and believes he or she is the center of the universe. It is also in this stage

that the child believes inanimate objects have life within, a concept known as animism. The child believes that punishment for bad deeds is inevitable.

3. The **Concrete (Operational) Stage** occurs from ages 7 to 11 years, when the child begins to understand how the world operates. The child comes to understand the concept of cause and effect and that actions and resultant consequences may be avoidable or reversible. Object permanence developed in the sensorimotor stage is enhanced with the addition of object equivalence. The child now understands the volume of the solid ice cube is equal to the water in its melted state.

4. The **Formal (Abstract) Stage** occurs at 11 years of age and projects throughout the rest of the individual's life. In this stage abstract concepts and the concept of probabilities are understood.

Erik Homburg Erikson's Stages of Development. Erik Homburg Erikson divided human development into 8 stages, the first 5 of which correlate with those of Freud and Piaget. These stages deal with the development of psychosocial maturational skills.

1. The **Trust Versus Mistrust** stage occurs in the infant from 0 to 1 year old. The child is dependent on caregivers and learns to trust the caregivers who provide food and protection. The child begins to learn mistrust of dangerous situations such as falling from high places.

2. The **Autonomy Versus Shame and Doubt** stage occurs in the toddler from ages 1 to 3 years and includes the process of toilet training. The child is conflicted by feelings of shame for his or her body and body products and is doubtful of his or her ability to function independently. At the same time, the child wants to develop autonomy.

3. The **Initiative Versus Guilt** stage occurs in the preschooler at ages 4 through 6 years. The child regains a sense of independence and competence which may be accompanied by guilt at not needing the parents as much. At this stage, Erikson postulated, the child begins to feel some regret for actions he or she has taken.

4. The **Industry Versus Inferiority** stage is from 7 to 11 years of age, when the child begins to work on extended projects at home and at school. This initiates a sense of successful task completion. If unable to complete projects successfully, feelings of inferiority and failure may develop.

5. The **Identity Versus Role Confusion** stage occurs in adolescence from 11 to 21 years with the individual playing many roles and seeking a comfort level in these different roles. The adolescent uses this time to discover himself or herself, testing the waters of different peer groups and identities and adopting different styles of dress.

ADOLESCENCE

Adolescence is a period marked by changes in biology, intellect, cognition, and social interaction. There is a difference between being an adolescent and being a teenager. Individuals reach adolescence at the age of 11 years and cease being an adolescent at 21 years. This is somewhat different from the designation of teenager, which begins at 13 years and ends after 19 years of age.

While children universally move into adolescence automatically, most cultures have rites of passage when children become teenagers. In the non-industrialized cultures, boys were once expected to engage in demonstrations of strength and courage as a means of becoming a man at the age of 13 years. In some cultures, girls became eligible for marriage and childbearing at the age of 13 years.

Adolescence is marked by physical changes in the body. Internal chemicals, hormones, begin to flow, heralding the onset of puberty. In boys the onset of the secondary characteristics of the deepening voice, the growth of visible facial hair, and the lengthening of the bones of the arms and legs is stimulated by the new surge of testosterone; testosterone is thought to underlie impulsive and aggressive behavior. In girls the change in body shape as well as the onset of menarche, is produced by the release of estradiol; from menarche to menopause, rising and lowering levels of estradiol affect mood.

These sex steroids are responsible for the primary and secondary sexual characteristics in men and women. It is the maturation of the hypothalamic-pituitary-adrenal-gonadal axis that puts this into motion. The primary sexual characteristics are related to the external genitalia and the reproductive organs responsible for procreation. The secondary sexual characteristics are the gender signposts. These are most recognizably enlarged breasts and hips in women and facial hair and lowering of the voice in men.

The age of onset of this new self varies from adolescent to adolescent. The onset of puberty tends to occur 1 to 1.5 years earlier in girls than in boys. For girls the average onset of puberty is at age 11 and ranges from age 8 to 13 years. The average age of onset for boys coincides with the worldwide age of passage of 13 years old. The range in boys is from age 10 to 14 years. On average, onset of menarche for girls occurs approximately 1.5 years earlier now than in the 1920s, when it began at age 14.5 years. The onset of menarche, or even the continuation of the menstrual cycle, can be adversely impacted by poor nutrition, excessive exercise, and/or psychological trauma and stress. The eating disorder anorexia nervosa serves as the prototype of lack of nutrition or excessive exercise, halting the menstrual cycle (see Eating Disorders on page 128).

The Stages of Adolescence

Early Adolescence
- Concerns about puberty
- Concrete thought processes
- Seeking independence
- Unisex peer group

Early adolescence occurs from age 11 to 14 years. The youngster is emerging from Freud's latency stage, as if a flower waiting to bloom. The flower awaits pollination by the release of the steroidal hormones. The child begins to experience changes in his or her body in ways he or she could never have imagined. The girl begins the menstrual cycles she will experience until the onset of menopause. The boy begins his journey into physical adult maleness with surges of testosterone and will begin to experience erections and nocturnal emissions that occur during sleep.

In this stage of development, the adolescent experiences unrealistic emotional fantasies or "crushes" on unobtainable love objects, such as movie, sports, and music stars. The early adolescent engages in hero worship and typically has older individuals, eg, teachers or friends' parents, as objects of emotional infatuation. The peer group ordinarily consists of members of the same sex. Boys most often belong to a group, and girls tend to have 2 or 3 best friends. The group or best friends share common dress patterns and often similar hairstyles. The youth engage in similar interests and ritualized activities. There is a strong sense of peer pressure. The personal superego, the adolescent's conscience, gives way to the sway of the group or best friends. To the adult's oft-asked question, "If your friends climbed onto the roof and jumped off, would you do that, too?" there would be a resounding affirmative answer. The early adolescent provides vague and unrealistic answers when asked about future plans.

Middle Adolescence
- Ambivalence about separating from family/parents
- Beginning heterosexual relationships/peer group
- Beginning of formal operational thought processes
- Sexual experimentation

This stage of adolescent development occurs from 14 to 17 years of age. During this stage, love objects begin to move closer to the adolescent's own age. While closer in age, the love object is often still an unobtainable fantasy: perhaps the cheerleader or the captain of the football team. In this stage, many adolescents begin experimentation with adult sexual behavior (Box 1). It is currently believed that the first sexual intercourse occurs around the age of 16 years for both men and women. At this stage, adolescents may also engage in same-sex experimentation that may lead the adolescent to recognize his or her sexual orientation as being lifelong same-sexed. During middle adolescence, the previous groups and best friends that were all boys and all girls give way to heterosexual peer groups, opening the door for dating. A key characteristic of middle adolescent sexuality is that one's partner is viewed as a "sex object," and both sexes perceive the dating relationship as affording social gain. If asked about future plans, the middle adolescent will be more focused than in early adolescence; however, the response may still be relatively unrealistic. The plans are viewed by the adolescent more as an escape from home or in over-glamorous terms.

Late Adolescence
- Beginning to formulate career plans
- Idealism
- Increasing abilities of abstraction
- Intimate relationships take precedence over the peer group

This stage occurs from 17 to 21 years of age. The late adolescent develops the capacity for true intimacy, the ability to care deeply for another person without exploiting that individual or viewing him or her as a vehicle for social gain. The adolescent begins to develop a clearer picture of his or her identity. Piaget spoke of the cognitive development of formal operations. Thinking becomes abstract, concepts form, and the individual becomes future-oriented.

Erikson viewed adolescence as working through the task of ego identity to discover who one is and where one is going. He highlighted identity versus role

Box 1. An Hypothesis with Regard to Adolescent Depression, Sexuality, and Cigarettes

Typically, the depressed adult will experience a decrease in libido and a loss of interest in sexual activity or intimacy. Often this is quite the opposite in adolescent depression, in which an increase in libido and sexual activity occurs. Just as adolescents and adults often self-medicate depression and other mental illnesses with legal and illegal substances, so too might adolescents self-medicate depression with increased sexual activity.

A decrease in the neurotransmitter dopamine may be responsible for depression in many individuals. By engaging in sexual activity, the adolescent receives a neuronal release of dopamine, temporarily enhancing mood. Sexual activity creates the self-perception of being more desirable, resulting in enhanced self-esteem. Enhanced self-esteem improves mood.

The role of dopamine may also help explain adolescent use of cigarettes. As the nicotine passes across the alveolar-blood barrier to the blood-brain barrier and into the central nervous system, there is a release of dopamine in the brain. This nicotine-induced dopamine release serves to medicate the depression.

confusion. Throughout the stages of adolescence, the individual tries on different uniforms of thought and dress. In late adolescence the individual has either brought things together to possess a secure sense of self (identity) or has not succeeded in developing a cohesive sense of self or self-awareness, resulting in identity diffusion and confusion.

As mentioned earlier, in early adolescence, peer pressure replaces the superego. By late adolescence, a renewed, matured superego appears. At this stage, the superego is inflexible and the concept of what is right and wrong is etched in stone. It is not until the late adolescent shifts into adulthood that the superego develops new flexibility. When the young adult needs to make a living, black and white give way to gray. When late adolescents find themselves legally bound by contracts, needing to buy car insurance, paying rent, repaying college loans, and starting their first potentially permanent job, the concept of compromise becomes very real. The late adolescent learns to go along to get along in the daily workforce.

Relationships shed their superficiality (Figure 1). True intimacy ensues and marriage may occur. When asked about future plans, the late adolescent either has fixed realistic plans or is truly unsure and seeks counsel. Adolescents who struggle with the decision-making process and eventually pursue what they want rather than what others want for them are more likely to achieve satisfaction in their lives.

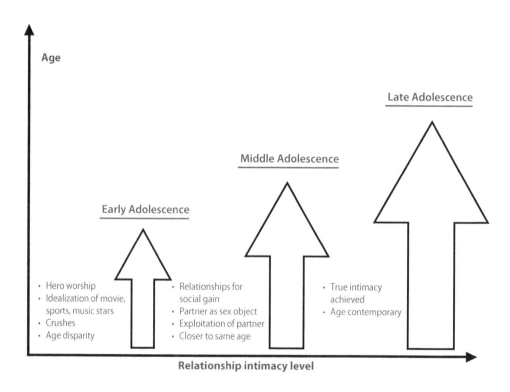

Figure 1. Realistic Intimacy Increases with Increasing Age Throughout Adolescence

DISORDERS OF CHILDHOOD AND ADOLESCENCE

Note: Before initiating any therapy, the clinician should obtain informed consent from the patient, parent, or guardian (see Appendix 1).

When the clinician assesses children and adolescents for psychiatric disturbance, the usual and customary triad of mood disorder, anxiety disorder, and thought disorder serves as the first component of assessment (Box 2). However, the assessment then broadens to include additional disorders commonly seen in children and adolescents:

- Attention-deficit hyperactivity disorder (and its spectrum of oppositional defiant disorder and conduct disorder)
- Developmental disorders (the autistic spectrum disorders)
- Elimination disorders (enuresis and encopresis)
- Eating disorders (anorexia nervosa, bulimia nervosa)
- Substance abuse and dependence (especially in adolescence and late adolescence)
- Tic disorders (Tourette's Disorder)

Box 2. Guidelines for Interviewing Adolescents

- Assess transference and countertransference issues
- Be nonjudgmental and remain objective
- Establish rapport
- Explain confidentiality
- Facilitate insight formation by the adolescent
- Interview the adolescent independent of his or her parents
- Obtain data

Topics to Assess
- Family issues
- Mood
- Past physical and sexual abuse
- Peer group
- School
- Self-esteem
- Sexual activity
- Substance usage
- Suicidal ideations and attempts

Attention-Deficit/Hyperactivity Disorder

Attention-deficit hyperactivity disorder (ADHD) is the psychiatric disease state most often diagnosed in childhood. It is a condition highlighted by heightened motor activity, disturbance in focus and concentration, or a combination of the two. Only recently has ADHD been diagnosed in adults and treatment regimens developed. It is understood today that 30% to 60% of those diagnosed with ADHD in childhood will persist with some form of the condition throughout their lifetime (see Chapter 8).

Autistic Spectrum Disorders

For some children and adolescents, behavioral disturbances are due to disruption in reading social cues and to an inability to connect socially with others. Some of these young people are unable to communicate verbally and those who can communicate verbally may demonstrate disturbances in voice modulation and amplitude.

Children with Autistic Disorder. These children demonstrate a paucity of social interaction and verbal skills very early in development. This disorder is diagnosed by 3 years of age. The individual will continue to demonstrate rigidity in behavior patterns, with a restricted repertoire of interests and activities. Autistic children whose routines are disrupted may become very agitated. Autistic children perform repetitive self-stimulatory behaviors, which may be seen as stereotypic movements and/or noises. While 70% of these children also experience mental retardation, 30% have either normal or above normal intelligence. Hand flapping and toe-walking are characteristic of the Autistic child.

Children with Asperger's Disorder. These children have difficulty receiving, interpreting, and acting on social cues. Individuals with Asperger's disorder do not respond well to change in routine. They may seem rigid or "oppositional and defiant" when in fact they are demonstrating their difficulty understanding social cues and customs, as well as their inability to adapt to immediate change in a given social or educational situation. Another feature is dysprosody, which is an eccentricity of speech. The speech in individuals with Asperger's disorder presents in a flat, monotone pattern, often with an odd pitch to it. The individual demonstrates neither animation nor inflection in his or her speech.

Viewed on a spectrum or continuum, autistic disorder is at the extreme of inability to engage others socially, inability to read social cues, and more often than not an inability to communicate verbally. Asperger's disorder is at the other end of the autistic spectrum—the individual is able to communicate verbally and often shows increased intellectual capacity, yet is unable to successfully understand social cues and becomes socially isolated because of eccentric behaviors (Figure 2).

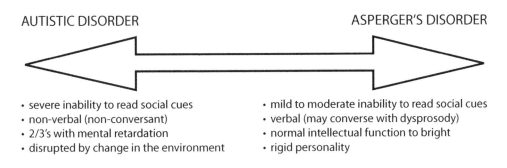

AUTISTIC DISORDER

ASPERGER'S DISORDER

- severe inability to read social cues
- non-verbal (non-conversant)
- 2/3's with mental retardation
- disrupted by change in the environment

- mild to moderate inability to read social cues
- verbal (may converse with dysprosody)
- normal intellectual function to bright
- rigid personality

Figure 2. The Autistic Spectrum

Elimination Disorders

A key component of a child's developmental process is control over bowel and bladder function. This control involves physical, psychological, and social factors. The development of bowel and bladder control is a process that evolves as the child matures.

Bowel and bladder control development follows a typical pattern. First, the child attains nighttime fecal control. Second, the child attains daytime fecal control. Third, the child attains daytime bladder control, and finally, the child attains nighttime bladder control.

The process of acquiring control is referred to as toilet training. Many factors influence toilet training including:

- Cultural factors
- Intellectual capacity
- Physiological factors
- Psychological interactions between the child and the parents
- Social maturity

Two elimination disorders, encopresis and enuresis, are included in the *Diagnostic and Statistical Manual of Mental Disorders, 4th Edition-TR.*

Encopresis. Encopresis is defined as the passage of fecal material in inappropriate places and/or at inappropriate times at least once per month for 3 consecutive months. This release of fecal material may be either voluntary or involuntary. To qualify for the diagnosis of encopresis, the child must be at least 4 years old either chronologically or in developmental equivalence.

In the industrialized nations, 95% of children achieve bowel control by the age of 4 years and 99% by age 5. Encopresis is almost nonexistent by age 16 years. Encopresis occurs more often in boys than in girls:

- Age 7 to 8 years – frequency is 1.5% in boys, 0.5% in girls
- Age 10 to 12 years – frequency is 1.3% in boys, 0.3% in girls

Encopresis has 3 possible underlying causes. The first is developmental, that is, the parents have not initiated toilet training in a timely fashion. A second cause is emotional as the child engages in a battle with the parents over autonomy and control. Finally, there may be a physiological cause. The child may suffer from incompetent sphincter control or lack the necessary nerve plexuses responsible for the voiding process (Box 3)

Children may choose to withhold defecation because of issues of control and self-esteem, anxiety, or painful defecation. In these instances, psychogenic megacolon occurs. Psychogenic megacolon results from the accumulation of fecal material in the colon, leading to distention of the colon. It becomes dilated and over time the child may no longer sense the signals indicating the need to defecate. This can lead to liquid stool pressing around the fecal obstruction and leaking out (overflow fecal incontinence). Anxiety can lead to diarrhea and the inability to control fecal passage as well.

When encopresis occurs, laboratory testing should be performed to identify and eliminate physical causes. Typical tests include:

- Abdominal x-ray to assess level of colonic stool
- Rectal examination
- Test for sphincter tone
- Test for Hirschsprung's disease

Box 3. Hirschsprung's Disease

Also known as congenital megacolon, Hirschsprung's disease involves an absence of the Meissner and Auerbach autonomic plexuses in the wall of the bowel, typically limited to the area of the colon. This results in either lack of digestive motility or abnormal digestive motility, causing partial or complete obstruction of the bowel as intestinal contents accumulate and create a massive dilation of the occluded section of bowel.

The child will present with obstipation, distention, and vomiting. If the motility is abnormal rather than absent, the child may experience intermittent constipation with alternating bouts of diarrhea. Depending on the severity of the disturbance, mild cases will often not be diagnosed until later in infancy. Early diagnosis helps to avoid the potential for toxic enterocolitis, which results from bacterial overgrowth in the small intestine and resultant production of bacterial toxins. These toxins cause explosive diarrhea with significant fluid loss, dehydration, and possible death. In older infants, the disturbance in bowel motility may result in anorexia, lack of the physiologic urge to defecate, visible peristalsis, a palpable colon, and on examination, an empty rectal vault. Infants with Hirschsprung's disease may demonstrate failure to thrive.

A barium enema reveals the colon to be dilated proximal to the site of the obstruction, and a narrowing of the distal segment, which lacks normal nerve plexus innervations. In newborns, the barium enema may not be diagnostic of toxic megacolon. Rectal biopsy provides the definitive diagnosis. Absence of the nerve ganglia is definitive of Hirschsprung's disease. Treatment is resection of the complete aganglionic portion of the colon.

If no physical cause is found, then treatment should focus on psychological causes and may include:

- Hypnosis
- Laxatives
- Psychotherapy/family therapy
- Reward/behavioral therapy
- Stool softeners

Enuresis. Enuresis is defined as the repeated voiding of urine into the bed linens or clothing at least twice a week for 3 or more months. To receive this diagnosis, the child must have reached the chronological or developmental age of 5 years. At age 2 years, 82% of children do not yet have full control of their bladder. By age 5, the percentage drops to 7%. The loss of urine in enuresis can be either voluntary or involuntary.

When diagnosing enuresis, the clinician should first rule out physiological causes, which include:

- Diabetes mellitus, diabetes insipidus
- Disturbances of sleep and/or consciousness, eg, intoxication, seizures, and sleepwalking disturbance
- Genitourinary disorders, which may be infectious, neurologic, or structural, eg, cystitis, obstructive uropathy, and spina bifida occulta
- Medication side effects, eg, Mellaril (thioridazine)

Enuresis is usually self-limited. Relapses of enuretic episodes are not uncommon, beginning between ages 5 and 8 years. If enuresis returns during adulthood, organic causes must be investigated.

The famous Isle of Wight study is the quintessential work with regard to the epidemiology and prognosis of enuresis. This study reported 15.2% of 7-year-old boys were enuretic occasionally and 6.7% were enuretic at least once a week; 3.3% of 7-year-old girls experienced enuresis at least once a week. The study reported the overall prevalence of enuresis to be 3% by age 10 years. The rate drops for teenagers in whom a prevalence of 1.5% has been reported for 14-year-olds.

Approximately 75% of children with enuresis have a first-degree relative who is or was enuretic. In some cases, the child's bladder capacity is normal when anesthetized; however, functionally it has a smaller capacity. Thus, the child feels a need to void when the bladder is filled with only a small amount of urine. Other children appear to have a lower-than-needed level of nighttime antidiuretic hormone, leading to higher nighttime urine output.

There has been much debate as to whether the child's sleep patterns are involved. Some experts argue these children have normal sleep architecture. Many clinicians, however, report mothers describing their child as experiencing a deeper than normal sleep, so their child is unaware of voiding cues.

- **Treatment of Enuresis**. Classic conditioning has been used in the past and continues to be used, involving a pad and a buzzer that sounds an alarm when the pad becomes wet. Reward/behavior programs are utilized as well.

Pharmacotherapy has also proven effective using Tofranil (imipramine) or DDAVP (desmopressin acetate) given at bedtime. Imipramine dosing may begin at 10 mg by mouth. In some children, this may be increased to as much as 200 mg at bedtime via slow upward titration to effectiveness. A pre-treatment electrocardiogram (ECG) is appropriate, and serum levels should be evaluated if the dosing regimen exceeds 40 mg. Another popular medication is DDAVP (desmopressin acetate), available as a nasal spray or a tablet. It is dosed as 0.1 to 0.4 mg per night. Once the enuresis is under control, discontinuing either medication may result in a return of symptoms, necessitating the re-initiation of the medication.

Hypnosis has shown benefit in treating enuretic episodes in some children. When used for nighttime bladder control, its effectiveness may result from the child's enhanced ability to sense physiologic cues of bladder fullness. Although not fully understood, hypnosis may assist the child in awakening from sleep at appropriate times to respond to the physiologic cues.

Enuresis is ego-dystonic for children, as well as socially limiting. Engaging the child and the family in therapy is an important component to remove the stigma, calm anxiety, and relieve the condition.

Anxious School Refusal/School Phobia (Separation Anxiety)

Hypothetical Case. Amanda is a 13-year-old female whose family recently moved from a small rural community to a larger urban center. Amanda changed from a school with 95 students to one with 275 students. She could no longer walk 3 blocks to school and now must ride on a school bus 30 minutes each way to reach her new school. Two weeks into the new school term, she complained of stomachaches in the morning and told her mother she did not feel she could go to school. Thinking she had a mild stomach virus, her mother allowed her to stay home. On the third day at home, her mother was concerned and took Amanda to their family physician to assess her stomachaches, nausea, vomiting, and diarrhea. Following evaluation, the physician sent her home, suggesting "Maybe it's something she ate or a stomach virus; let's reassess her in a couple of days if this persists." The next morning Amanda felt better, so her mom sent her to school, in spite of the teen seeming a bit anxious. On the bus, she started to feel uneasy; before arriving at school, she began to breathe quickly and experience excessive perspiration and a more rapid heart rate. Once at school, she was sent to the school nurse, who called the girl's mother to take her home. Amanda was seen again by the family physician and assessed according to the following diagnostic tree of rule-outs and rule-ins, any of which can mimic anxiety disorder:

- Caffeinism
- Cardiac dysrhythmias
- Hyperthyroidism
- Hypoglycemic episodes
- Migraine headache
- Peptic ulcer disease
- Pheochromocytoma
- Seizure disorder
- Substance abuse/medication reaction

She was also assessed for a history of taking any of the following types of medications, which can simulate an anxiety response:

- Antiasthmatics
- Antihistamines
- Antipsychotics (akathisia) [for unknown reasons, Haldol (haloperidol) and Orap (pimozide) can cause a school-phobia phenomenon in a small subset of children]
- Nonprescription preparations including diet pills and cold remedies
- Serotonin selective reuptake inhibitors (SSRIs)
- Steroids
- Sympathomimetics

Having ruled out organic causes and medication side effects as the causative agent, the family physician suspected Amanda was suffering from an anxiety disorder. As discussed in Chapter 2, these range from acute stress disorder to phobias. In children and adolescents, separation anxiety disorder/school phobia is a common anxiety disorder.

Amanda feels sick in the morning when it is time to go to school. If she stays home from school, she starts to feel better. She will do anything not to go to school. She will become physically ill, she will cry, she will lock herself in the bathroom when it is time to catch the bus. Amanda has anxious school refusal/ school phobia. Estimates range from 3 to 17 cases per 1000 school children each year, with equal prevalence in males and females.

Clinical Features. As noted in the hypothetical case, the school-refusing child not only fears going to school, he or she also resists going to school, and will attempt to remain at home during school hours. A child with anxious school refusal/school phobia generally exhibits a set of classic symptoms:

- The child has vague or specific somatic complaints such as headache, stomachache, nausea, vomiting, and/or diarrhea.
- Once on the way to school, the child becomes extremely anxious and resists going into the school building.
- If the child is allowed to stay home, the symptoms abate.
- The child does not complain of symptoms on weekends.
- The child is fine after normal school hours have ended.

Often the child will present logical reasons for not attending school, such as a teacher (or all the teachers) is being unfair; the child is being threatened by a bully at school; or the child is embarrassed to publicly shower, wear revealing gym clothes, or suffer the indignities in the locker room of physical education class.

While the reality of these reasons typically evaporates after investigation, sometimes the reasons prove valid. In such cases, once the situation is corrected, the school refusal may resolve. In most instances, the cited apprehension is merely a rationalization of a deeply rooted inner anxiety; environmental manipulations involving changes in schools, classes, neighborhoods, and/or teachers often prove ineffective in relieving the anxiety. As children move from the latency stage (6–11 years) into early and middle adolescence (11–17 years), issues of body form become real, and concerns of public showering and revealing clothing need to be assessed.

The onset of anxious school refusal/school phobia or an exacerbation of an ongoing previously remitted school refusal often occurs after stressful events, such as a brief illness, a vacation, a change in residence, a change of school, the weekend, or a trauma (eg, a death, family loss, or family upheaval that heightens the child's/family's level of anxiety).

Change is unsettling for many children, adolescents, and adults. In the child with the propensity for anxious school refusal/school phobia, any change in routine can be anxiety provoking and present as increased fear of leaving the household to attend school. Thus, as change begets anxiety, the onset (or re-onset) of anxiety can ignite or re-ignite anxious school refusal/school phobia. The underlying anxiety that presents as anxious school refusal/school phobia is actually separation anxiety.

Separation Anxiety. When first attending preschool or nursery school, children commonly experience initial anxiety. With parental, teacher, and peer support, most children adapt to the experience. On the other hand, some children have persistent separation difficulties. If the parent (most often the mother or other custodial adult) also experiences anxiety about the separation, this resonates between the child and the parent and is magnified. At this developmental stage, the young child expresses his or her "clinginess" openly and directly without converting the feelings of anxiety into physical discomfort and complaint (somatization).

The latency stage (6–11 years) school-refusing child does not express the dependent desire openly and may not consciously recognize this dependency need. Instead the child may enlist the unconscious defenses of avoidance, displacement, and somatization in dealing with the anxiety over the availability of the attachment figures (usually the parents).

In adolescence there is a strong developmental push toward separation and independence. If school refusal is first diagnosed in the period of early adolescence (11–14 years) or middle adolescence (14–17 years), a careful history will usually reveal a long series of past school absences with implicit collusion by the parent(s) in the child's separation avoidance.

Some experts believe there might be a genetic component, in that one parent may have experienced separation anxiety as a child or suffers from agoraphobia. Psychiatric disorders often occur in multiple generations of a family and appear to be genetically transmitted. Anxiety disorder found in a family may manifest in a child as separation anxiety, which leads to anxious school refusal/school phobia. Often children will experience a medication-induced anxious school refusal/school phobia when taking either haloperidol or pimozide. It is unclear what leads to these dopamine-blocking medications causing an anxiety phenomenon; however, discontinuation of the medication results in remission of the anxious school refusal/school phobia symptoms.

Treatment. The longer the child stays home, the more difficult it becomes to return to school (Box 4). The child becomes more isolated from friends, homework accumulates, and the child's unresolved fears grow in his or her imagination. Until the child and family actively confront this separation anxiety, the conflicts concerning school attendance and separation cannot be resolved. Family therapy is an integral part of the therapeutic approach. Even after the child has returned to school, it is important to continue treatment. Relapses are common, and often the anxiety may take some other symptomatic form.

Box 4. Dr. Goldman's Reverse Re-entry Technique

A method to re-introduce a child with school phobia into the classroom is to have the child attend just one class hour of school initially, slowly "titrating" upward the amount of time spent at school. The Reverse Reentry Technique has the child start the school day during the last class session of the day. Once the student demonstrates comfort with that time frame, he or she attends the last 2 classes. As the student gains comfort with each additional hour, another hour is added until the student returns to a full day of classes. This technique succeeds for 3 reasons. First, the student realizes that at the end of the first hour of re-entry, he or she will be going home. Second, as all the other students are also leaving school at the end of that class, the student does not stand out for leaving for home. Third, the day seems less overwhelming if the student is not coming in first hour and leaving early, seeing the "whole day" ahead of him or her. The student is confronted by a manageable block of time.

- **Pharmacotherapy**. Several approaches have shown benefit. A traditional approach has been the tricyclic antidepressants. Imipramine helps to calm the individual's anxiety, as well as improve mood. As a tricyclic antidepressant, it also facilitates sleep at night as a result of its sedating side effect. Currently, imipramine is approved by the US Food and Drug Administration (FDA) to treat only depression in children, so its use to treat anxiety is off-label. Because of its potential side effect of slowing electrical conduction through the cardiac muscle, the clinician should obtain a baseline ECG prior to initiation and a follow-up ECG after the tricyclic antidepressant medication has been initiated. If the individual has any prior existing cardiac conduction abnormalities, it is prudent not to initiate a tricyclic antidepressant. Serum levels of imipramine should also be assessed for safety.

Imipramine's cousin, Anafranil (clomipramine), is another beneficial medication, as it has the properties of imipramine with the added benefit of the anti-obsessional quality secondary to the enhanced inhibition of the presynaptic reuptake transport pump for serotonin. While SSRIs have proven beneficial in treating anxiety in both children and adults, currently none has been approved for this use in children. Prozac (fluoxetine) is FDA approved to treat depression in children and, along with Zoloft (sertraline) and Anafranil (clomipramine), to treat pediatric obsessive-compulsive disorder. Chapter 2 highlights the SSRIs that are effective in treating various adult anxieties; some of these medications may be prescribed off-label in children as well.

The benzodiazepines are beneficial for short-term use to calm an immediate episode of anxiety. Xanax (alprazolam) has the most rapid onset with a very short half-life.

Eating Disorders

Just as depression occurs more often in women than men, so too the eating disorders occur more often in women than in men. Eating disorders are estimated to occur 10 to 20 times more frequently in women. Bulimia nervosa occurs more frequently than anorexia nervosa, and up to 40% of college women report they have engaged in at least 1 episode of binge eating followed by self-induced vomiting.

For many individuals, the only component of their lives they feel is controllable is diet. They will control what goes in and what comes out via food restriction, purging from the top end of the alimentary tract by self-induced vomiting, or purging from the bottom end of the alimentary tract by laxative abuse. Alternatively, there may be "calorie purging" through excessive exercise.

While anorexia nervosa is classically associated with food restriction and "exercise purging" and bulimia nervosa is associated with self-induced vomiting, the *Diagnostic and Statistical Manual of Mental Disorders, 4th Edition-TR* lists 2 types of anorexia nervosa, restricting type and binge eating/purging type. The rule of thumb is to still think of anorexia nervosa as restricting and bulimia nervosa as binge eating followed by purging. The key to distinguishing anorexia nervosa from bulimia nervosa is the individual's actual body weight. The individual with anorexia nervosa is at least 15% below ideal body weight, while the individual with bulimia nervosa is usually at or above ideal body weight.

Because of the prevalence of these conditions in women, clinicians should maintain a healthy index of suspicion when interviewing females. Often at the core of eating disorders are peer pressure and social "norms" for thinness, dating "desirability," and chic fashion. These combine with family problems, issues of control, self-identity confusion, or sexual abuse.

In assessing the individual for an eating disorder, questions about self-perception of body image are very important. The individual's misperception may be so dramatic that she or he may have what would seem to be a delusional disorder, known as body dysmorphic disorder. They have a fixed false perception of their body that is dramatically at odds with an objective perspective of their appearance.

Individuals with anorexia nervosa typically are more ingrained in their illness and feel their disorder is ego-syntonic, meaning it allows them to feel better about themselves. They feel a greater sense of control over their lives and their environment. Their food restriction and loss of weight actually bring them a sense of accomplishment. On the other hand, those suffering from bulimia nervosa usually feel the binge-eating episodes and the resulting purging episodes are ego-dystonic, eliciting guilt and shame. These individuals do not feel good about themselves and will seek help from a therapist far more often than do those suffering from anorexia nervosa.

The food restriction of anorexia nervosa adversely impacts nutrition and growth. It can disrupt bone development, skin and hair production, and growth; it can retard or cause cessation of the menstrual cycle; and it can damage cardiac tissue. Extreme weight loss can cause bradycardia, edema, lanugo hair, hypotension, and hypothermia. Self-induced vomiting can disrupt electrolyte balance, adversely impacting cardiac function; it can damage the epithelium of the esophagus, erode the enamel of the teeth, and cause dehydration, hyperamylasemia, hypochloremic alkalosis, hypokalemia, and hypomagnesemia. Although bulimia nervosa tends to have a better course and prognosis than anorexia nervosa, both disorders can result in death.

When an eating disorder is suspected, the physical examination is an important component to assess the individual's physical well-being. The clinician should assess nutrition and ask questions about appetite and eating habits. Women should be asked about their menstrual cycle and flow. The physical examination should include measurements of height and weight, heart rate, and blood pressure. Laboratory tests should check for electrolyte balance and glucose levels. Skin, hair, nails, mouth, and teeth should be examined and an ECG performed. Bowel habits should be assessed. The results of these usual and customary components of the physical examination are likely to be found to be outside of the normal limits in individuals with eating disorders.

The physical examination and laboratory tests provide important information in these psychiatric disorders. In the examination, clinicians should particularly note any combination of the following:

- Abnormal disruption in height and weight
- Abrasion of the first 2 knuckles of either hand secondary to self-induced vomiting (the knuckles rub against the upper front teeth in the process)
- Bradycardia (detected by feeling the pulse and heart rate when taking vital signs)
- Erosion of the enamel on the backside of the teeth
- Hair loss
- Hypotension (due to hypovolemia)
- Hypothermia (revealed by oral temperature when taking vital signs)
- Increase in dental caries
- Lack of menses (in females)
- Lanugo hair
- Tenting of the skin due to dehydration

Laboratory results may reveal any of a series of abnormalities, including:

- ECG irregularities
- Hyperamylasemia
- Hypochloremia
- Hypokalemia
- Hypomagnesemia

The outcome in individuals with anorexia nervosa is variable, with any of the following possible:

- A spontaneous recovery
- A treatment responsive course
- A waxing and waning course
- Death (statistics range from 5% to 18%)

The outcome for individuals with bulimia nervosa, while variable, is usually better than for those with anorexia nervosa and typically involves a waxing and waning course with remissions and exacerbations. Treatment for both conditions involves:

- Full medical assessment
- Hospitalization
- Pharmacologic intervention
- Psychotherapy

Pharmacologically, the serotonergic medications are typically the medications of choice. Of the SSRIs, Paxil (paroxetine) has the greatest potential for stimulating appetite and adding weight. A second-generation medication, Remeron (mirtazapine), will also stimulate appetite and increase weight, as it has an antihistaminergic moiety that is responsible for the appetite enhancement and weight gain. The lower the dose of mirtazapine, the greater the antihistaminergic impact. Thus, 15 mg is more sedating and more likely to increase weight than 30 mg, and 30 mg is more likely to do so than 45 mg.

The tricyclic antidepressant clomipramine is strongly serotonergic. As a tricyclic antidepressant, it has a greater potential for weight gain than the SSRIs. The antidepressant Wellbutrin (bupropion) IR/SR/XL should be avoided. It has the potential to lessen appetite and stimulate some weight loss. In addition, an early study found it had the potential to lower the seizure threshold when dosed above 450 mg per day, which could have adverse consequences in individuals with bulimia nervosa, who are already at greater risk of seizures because of electrolyte imbalance.

Tourette's Disorder

Tourette's disorder is a neurologic disorder, with onset before 18 years of age, in which the individual displays both motor and vocal tics. The motor and vocal tics need not occur concomitantly. While not a thought disorder or psychosis, Tourette's disorder is typically treated with antipsychotic medications. The key to the diagnosis is that the tics have persisted for more than 12 months and there has not been a tic-free period during that time for more than 3 consecutive months. The classical treatment approach for Tourette's disorder is haloperidol or pimozide, prescribed as 0.5 mg by mouth at bedtime initially, with upward titration as clinically indicated to 2 or 3 times a day. While these medications are still considered the gold standard for initial treatment, because of the potential side effects with the old-line typical antipsychotics, most practitioners today prescribe as first-line treatment the atypical antipsychotics, and use clonidine or Tenex (guanfacine), both alpha$_2$ agonists, as their second-line approach.

CHAPTER EIGHT

Attention-Deficit/ Hyperactivity Disorder

The diagnosis of attention-deficit/hyperactivity disorder (ADHD) as a disease state was first documented in 1902 by the British pediatrician George Frederic Still, who perceived it as a "defect in moral control." In the 1960s, Stella Chase coined the phrase *hyperactive child syndrome* and opened the door to the biological underpinning of ADHD. In 1980 the American Psychiatric Association (APA) gave the cluster of symptoms the new diagnostic name of attention-deficit disorder (ADD) with and without hyperactivity. In 1987, the APA renamed this medical condition attention-deficit/hyperactivity disorder, which is the current diagnostic term.

Three subtypes of ADHD have been delineated. The hyperactive type is synonymous with hyperactivity, impulsivity, and intrusiveness. These children are excessively active, climbing inappropriately on objects and having difficulty sitting still. They will not stay seated in the classroom or other environments. The hyperactive child interrupts others, speaks out of turn, and is unable to wait patiently in line.

In adulthood, these symptoms transform into a feeling of inner restlessness. Adults express a feeling of being overwhelmed. Because of their inner restlessness, they demonstrate a pervasive impatience, often completing others' sentences, for example, and not giving others the time to collect and complete their own thoughts.

The inattentive type of childhood ADHD brings on an inability to focus, making it difficult to organize homework and listen to teachers, parents, and friends. The inattentive type of ADHD morphs in adulthood into forgetfulness, difficulty managing time, and frequent distraction. The inattentiveness and restlessness in adulthood result in employment challenges and disruption in relationship stability.

The third subtype of ADHD is a combination that manifests itself in childhood with increased motor activity, increased impulsiveness, increased intrusion into

Box 1: ADHD Across the Life-Span: Childhood Through Adulthood

CHILDREN	ADOLESCENTS	ADULTS
"As if driven by a motor"	Inner restlessness	Inner restlessness
Intrusive into other's belongings and space	Difficulty organizing	Difficulty organizing
Interrupts others	Oppositional/Defiant behavior	Irritability
Difficulty waiting turn	Engages in risk-taking behaviors	Impulsive when making decisions
Easily distracted	Difficulty managing time	Difficulty managing time
Blurts out answers to questions	Low self-esteem	Low self-esteem
In constant motion in the classroom	Difficulty with focus and concentration	Difficulty with focus and concentration
Forgets books and assignments	Forgetful	Forgetful
Difficulty staying on task	Difficulty staying on task	Difficulty with planning ahead

ADHD for many is a life-long disease. While typically diagnosed in childhood, 30% to 60% of individuals will continue with its course throughout the entire lifespan. The hyperactivity of childhood morphs into restlessness in adolescence and adulthood. The difficulty with focus and concentration is a constant in ADHD throughout the lifespan. The inability to organize and plan remains constant. Difficulty judging time and planning ahead are evident in adolescence and adulthood. The constant correction, redirection, criticism, and reprimands lead to a decline in self-esteem and in the adolescent a reactive oppositional/defiant behavior. In the adult this is manifested in irritability and anger. Due to the decline in self-esteem, there may be a comorbid depression in adolescents and adults; the constant correction, redirection, criticism, and reprimands may also lead to comorbid depression in children. A common thread throughout the lifespan is a disruption in sleep patterns: circadian rhythm disruption. Some children and adolescents are able to maintain enough ego-strength and coping skills to succeed in school without being diagnosed and treated for their ADHD. It isn't until life stressors exceed their compensatory abilities that the symptoms and impairments become obvious. Graduation from high school and movement to college may tip the balance for some adolescents. Marriage and/or job promotion may be the culprit in tipping the balance for adults.

others' space and activities, difficulty focusing, difficulty concentrating, and difficulty managing time. The combined type of ADHD changes in adulthood into difficulty organizing, forgetfulness, mismanagement of time, and restlessness with work and relationships (Box 1).

COMORBIDITIES AND CONFOUNDERS IN ADHD

ADHD is a disorder that often occurs in conjunction with other psychiatric disorders. Morbidity relates to disturbance in daily life functioning; when several disorders occur together, they are termed *comorbid* or *comorbidities*. Illnesses that have symptoms similar to other illnesses and thus are easily confused or misdiagnosed for the other illness(es) are known as *confounders*. Often times the confounders can also be found along with a specific illness and hence meet the criteria as both a confounder and comorbidity. Below is a list of common confounders and comorbidities found with ADHD:

- Anxiety disorder
- Bipolar disorder
- Conduct disorder
- Depressive disorder
- Intermittent explosive disorder
- Obsessive-compulsive disorder
- Oppositional defiant disorder
- Post-traumatic stress disorder
- Sleep disorder(s)
- Substance abuse disorder
- Tourette's disorder

Anxiety Disorder

Children and adolescents with anxiety disorder often show fidgeting and nervous, non-productive activity that resembles inattention, hyperactivity, and inability to focus and complete tasks. It is important to assess the family history for anxiety disorder. Chapter 7 discusses the diagnosis and treatment of anxiety in children.

Bipolar Disorder

Distinguishing ADHD from bipolar disorder can be very difficult. Children with either disorder may exhibit inattentiveness, increased motor activity, impulsive behaviors, intrusive behaviors, aggressive behaviors, difficulty concentrating, and the appearance of racing thoughts. In some youngsters, ADHD may be the premorbid illness prior to the onset of bipolar disorder; and some researchers posit these 2 disorders may occur concomitantly. The key to accurately diagnosing bipolar disorder versus ADHD is a good family history and a careful assessment of the 6 neurovegetative functioning inventory indices (Chapter 1). If the clinician suspects comorbid bipolar disorder, the gold standard of treatment is a major mood stabilizer, as described in Chapter 1. Once mood is stabilized, then intervention for the ADHD is indicated. The gold standard for treating ADHD with medication is still the psychostimulants, especially the long-acting medications that provide smooth benefit without rebounding (see below). Rebounding from short-acting immediate-release psychostimulants is oftentimes misdiagnosed as or confused with bipolar disorder. In rebounding, individuals will display irritability, mood lability, crying, agitation, and increased disorganization. The clinician should monitor the times that parents report their child's symptoms, observing for a pattern. Do these symptoms occur the same time every day? Do they disappear on weekends if the medication is withheld?

Conduct Disorder

Conduct disorder is part of the ADHD continuum, with progression from ADHD to oppositional defiant disorder to conduct disorder to antisocial personality disorder. In conduct disorder, the individual has reached an age at which the once "tolerable" impulsivity and intrusiveness place the individual in contention with the law. Because the individual is no longer a child, he or she is at risk of legal consequences that will cause a downward spiral in the individual's social status. Conduct disorder is characterized by 3 behaviors, for which **ADD** is a suitable mnemonic:

- **A** = **A**ggressive behaviors
- **D** = **D**eceitful behaviors
- **D** = **D**estructive behaviors

The ADHD Continuum:

ADHD → Oppositional Defiant Disorder → Conduct Disorder $\xrightarrow{50\%}$ Antisocial Personality Disorder

Early intervention for ADHD is the key to preventing conduct disorder. Statistically 50% of those who progress to conduct disorder go on to develop antisocial personality disorder.

Depressive Disorder

Children and adolescents with ADHD are constantly corrected, redirected, criticized, and reprimanded. Because of this constant barrage, many children and adolescents stop hearing the comments describing bad behavior and start perceiving themselves to be bad people. This often leads to a decline in self-esteem with a resulting reactive depression, necessitating treatment for both depression and ADHD simultaneously, as described below.

Intermittent Explosive Disorder

Children, adolescents, and adults with intermittent explosive disorder react to situations with behaviors that are in excess of what would/should be a "usual and customary" response. Individuals demonstrate excessive anger and physical response. After the episode, they will often be remorseful and admit they exceeded appropriate behavioral response. If the individual has been taking a short-acting immediate-release psychostimulant, rebounding can result in intermittent explosive disorder–like symptoms, which can be relieved by prescribing a smooth, long-acting psychostimulant. If the individual truly has intermittent explosive disorder along with ADHD, stabilizing the explosive disorder first, then adding an extended-release psychostimulant is a balanced treatment approach.

Obsessive-Compulsive Disorder

Obsessive-compulsive disorder is an anxiety disorder, which often accompanies ADHD (a comorbidity) or can be confused with it (a confounder). Youngsters with obsessive-compulsive disorder are often driven to perform activities that appear as if they are impulsive or intrusive, when in reality they are anxiety-driven rituals. For example, a student may be unable to stay in his seat, as he gets up, walks into the hallway, turns around 3 times, hops on 1 foot 3 times, and returns to his seat. The teacher may see this as hyperactive behavior, when in reality it is an obsessive-compulsive disorder anxiety-driven ritual. Because a psychostimulant may exacerbate the obsessive-compulsive behaviors, it is important to make the correct diagnosis and then treat accordingly (see Chapter 2).

Oppositional Defiant Disorder

As described above, this disorder is an element in the ADHD continuum, usually thought to be the result of untreated or undertreated ADHD. Individuals who are not initiated in a pharmacologic and/or behavioral program will start to develop unconscious defense mechanisms to the constant redirections, corrections, criticisms, and reprimands that arise in response to their ADHD. This reaction to unconscious mechanisms in defense of ego develops into an oppositional style. This can become very disruptive to interactions between the student and teachers/faculty, between the child/adolescent and parents, and between the child/adolescent and peers. As they move from pre-adolescent into the teenage years, these individuals with oppositional defiant disorder may very easily and quickly shift into conduct disorder. Initiating therapy with medication and/or psychotherapy helps the child or adolescent develop the focus/concentration/skills to manage the ADHD and avoid progression to oppositional defiant disorder.

Post-Traumatic Stress Disorder

Children, adolescents, and adults who suffer from post-traumatic stress disorder may exhibit symptoms that are misdiagnosed as ADHD (a confounder). Anxiousness, disruption in concentration and focus, fidgeting, irritability, and mood lability/instability are very common for individuals with post-traumatic stress disorder. It is especially important for the clinician to take a complete history that includes an assessment for physical, emotional, sexual, and verbal abuse.

Sleep Disorders

Sleep disturbances are commonly reported in children with ADHD. The question arises: Does ADHD cause sleep disturbances or do sleep disturbances cause ADHD? The answer most likely is "yes" to both questions. It is currently the wisdom of child and adolescent psychiatry that ADHD is a multi-factorial disorder with multiple presentations of related symptoms. Sleep is one of these related symptoms. Some children with ADHD are unable to muster enough organization to go to sleep at night. For these youngsters, a small amount of short-acting, immediate-release psychostimulant proves beneficial if given 1 to 2 hours before bedtime. For other youngsters, it is important to assess whether the medication given during the day, late afternoon, or even early evening is the culprit itself for disturbing the sleep patterns. When children as well as adolescents and adults do not receive enough sleep during the night, focus, concentration, memory, and mood will be disrupted. Thus, before making the diagnosis of ADHD, it is important to assess the individual's sleep patterns and habits. A sleep study might be in order.

As in adults, children can suffer from obstructive sleep apnea/hypopnea syndrome (OSA/HS), which causes a decrease in needed oxygenation during sleep and disrupts the sleep cycles and benefit from sleep. These individuals may appear to have ADHD when in fact the symptoms may actually be the sequela of OSA/HS. Assessing sleep hygiene is important; a sleep study may be definitive.

Students should also be assessed for shift work sleep disorder, as many students do not have a traditional work/wake/sleep schedule (see Chapter 9).

Appendix 2 offers suggestions for diagnosing sleep disorders and inducing sleep.

Substance Abuse Disorder

In the past, it was said that introducing children to psychostimulant medications early in their lives predisposed them to substance abuse as adolescents. However, current research and medical practice have shown that treating ADHD as early as possible will actually help individuals avoid becoming substance abusers. When the impulsivity is treated early, thereby avoiding the transition to oppositional defiant disorder and conduct disorder, the child/adolescent will not be subjected to the barrage of criticisms and reprimands. Thus, he or she will avoid reactive depression and the adolescent will not need to self-medicate with illicit substances. Prescribing a long-acting medication avoids the buzz that children and adolescents may obtain from a short-acting, immediate-release psychostimulant, hence not conditioning the individual to look for a medication buzz as the key to success.

Tourette's Disorder

As noted in Chapter 7, Tourette's disorder manifests with motor and vocal tics: sudden, rapid, recurrent, nonrhythmic, stereotyped motor movements or vocalizations. While the motor and vocal tics do not have to occur concurrently, the individual must experience both for the diagnosis of Tourette's disorder to be made. The individual must not have a tic-free period of more than 3 consecutive months. Transient tic disorder is the diagnosis if the condition lasts for less than 1 year. Tic disorder not otherwise specified is the diagnosis made when the child/adolescent does not meet these criteria for Tourette's disorder. While the motor tics can be of any type, the most common is eye blinking. The vocal tics may occur as coughing, sniffing, snorting, throat clearing, or some other audible noise. Some individuals will demonstrate coprolalia (blurting out obscene words) and/or copropraxia (obscene gestures).

Motor and vocal tics are distressing to the individual with Tourette's disorder. While observers may misinterpret the individual's actions as behavioral disturbances, in fact, he or she is not volitionally engaging in these tic behaviors.

These individuals may be able to suppress the tics for a short period of time, sometimes up to 1 hour. However, it is as if the tics are "stored up," and after the hour of suppression, there will be a flurry of tics as if they are being released.

The treatment of choice for Tourette's disorder has been the dopamine-blocking typical antipsychotic medications such as Haldol (haloperidol) and Orap (pimozide) (see Chapter 3).

PRESCRIBING MEDICATION FOR ADHD

Note: Before initiating any therapy, the clinician should obtain informed consent from the individual, parent, or guardian (see Appendix 1).

The 2 distinctive components of ADHD are hyperactivity and inattention, and psychostimulant medications are the gold standard for treating both. While the inattention component will respond to both psychostimulant and non-psychostimulant medications, the hyperactivity and impulsivity of ADHD respond best to psychostimulant medications. As the choices of ADHD medications have become more numerous, combinations of medications have become popular to address specific components of the disease state. Psychostimulants are used concomitantly with alpha$_2$ agonists, atypical antipsychotic medications, and antiseizure medications. Often these combinations are employed if the child is manifesting aggressive behavior. With comorbid decreases in mood, antidepressant medications are initiated.

When psychostimulant medications are prescribed in children and adolescents, the clinician needs to carefully assess the amount and timing of the dose.

The Historical Short-Acting Psychostimulant Approach

Prior to the advent of the current long-acting psychostimulant medication treatments available for ADHD, the prevailing treatment gold standard was the short-acting, immediate-release psychostimulants. These medications were methylphenidate (MPH), amphetamine (AMP), and dextroamphetamine (dAMP) formulations. Successful use of these medications relied on the correct amount of medication given at the correct times. Typical short-acting mediations require approximately 45 to 60 minutes for their benefit to begin, with the length of the benefit of the short-acting medications varying from person to person and ranging from 2 to 4 hours. When the benefit starts to wear off, some youngsters experience a phenomenon known as rebounding (Figure 1). During rebounding, the child does not return to the pre-medicated state; rather he or she experiences an increase in agitation, disorganization, irritability, impulsivity, and/or inattention to a level far in excess of what it was at baseline without medication. When children rebound, their parents will usually report that "the medication doesn't work at all," when in reality it works, it just needs to be dosed more often to avoid the rebounding phenomenon. Historically, some youngsters were misdiagnosed with bipolar disorder because of the mood disruption caused by rebounding.

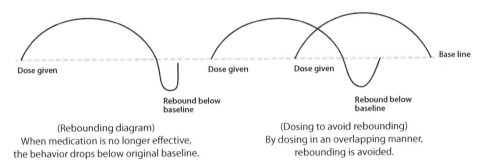

(Rebounding diagram)
When medication is no longer effective,
the behavior drops below original baseline.

(Dosing to avoid rebounding)
By dosing in an overlapping manner,
rebounding is avoided.

Figure 1. The Rebounding Phenomenon with Immediate-Release Psychostimulants

The Dosing Procedure of the Short-Acting, Immediate-Release Psycho-stimulants. The original approach consisted of writing a prescription for 5-mg tablets of MPH in a quantity sufficient for the parents to carry out the following regimen:

The child was initiated on one 5-mg tablet on Saturday morning and monitored from 8 AM until noon. The parents were to observe for (1) onset of medication; (2) duration of benefit; (3) offset of medication; and (4) possible rebounding/ side effects.

If no benefit occurred within the first 4 hours with the initial MPH 5-mg tablet, then after lunch the child was given 2 of the 5-mg tablets and the above 4-step monitoring process was again undertaken.

If no benefit accrued from the 10-mg dose, then on Sunday morning at 8 AM, 3 of the 5-mg tablets were given to the child. Again the 4-step monitoring process was followed. If no benefit accrued by noon, then after lunch 4 of the 5-mg tablets were given. Typically, if no benefit had accrued previously, by 20 mg there was usually benefit.

If the MPH proved ineffective, the next step was to initiate a similar trial of short-acting, immediate-release AMP/dAMP with the initial dose being 2.5 mg.

Once benefit was noted, the key was to observe for length of duration of the benefit. For some youngsters, each dose would provide 4 hours of benefit, for others only 2 hours of benefit was achieved. Doses must be scheduled to overlap to avoid rebounding. As the first dose was beginning to decline in benefit, the second dose was beginning to ramp upward so as to avoid rebounding and periods of being uncovered by medication benefit (see rebounding diagram above). Some youngsters benefited from dosing of the medication every 2 hours because of their rapid metabolizing of the medication (Box 2). MPH has a softer, gentler edge than AMP, with less appetite suppression and less mood lability and irritability than is generated by AMP. The US Food and Drug Administration (FDA) has approved dosing of MPH as 1 to 2 mg/kg; AMP is approved for 0.5 to 1 mg/kg.

The target for dosing of either MPH or AMP as a short-acting, immediate-release treatment approach was to prescribe the right amount to reach the threshold of benefit without overshooting that threshold. If the dose surpasses the necessary threshold of benefit, the individual is at risk for developing side effects, such as agitation, exacerbation of obsessive-compulsive disorder, headache, irritability, tachycardia, or tics.

Box 2. Calculating the Individual's Weight

Typically dosing of MPH, AMPs, dAMPs, and methamphetamines is clinically based on the individual's response to the medication as a result of his or her metabolic rate. Some individuals are rapid metabolizers, whose bodies utilize the medication very rapidly, thus needing either a larger dose or more frequent dosings to maintain benefit. The goal is to reach effectiveness without side effects. Calculating dosage as milligrams per kilogram of individual's weight provides the maximum dosing level. To obtain the individual's weight in kilograms, divide the individual's scale weight in pounds by 2.2. While most commonly the medications are not dosed by weight, it is the milligram per kilogram formula that ultimately provides the upper end or maximum dose [eg: 77 pounds ÷ 2.2 = 35kg].

The Long-Acting Psychostimulants

In 2000, a new medication was approved that changed the treatment of ADHD. Although MPH was its main ingredient, this new medication used a delivery system that allowed this active ingredient to be metered out throughout the day to provide full-day coverage with only morning dosing. The MPH is housed in a capsule that does not dissolve in the gastrointestinal tract. The capsule contains a small manufactured membrane that slowly moves upward, metering out the medication as it goes. Both in theory and in clinical reality, it provides smooth, all-day benefit. This medication is Concerta, which became the prototype for the long-acting, sustained-release psychostimulant ADHD medications that quickly followed in its footsteps.

Just as Prozac (fluoxetine) began the serotonin selective reuptake inhibitor (SSRI) revolution, Concerta began the long-acting psychostimulant medication revolution. The medication comes in capsule doses of 18, 27, 36, and 54 mg and is FDA approved to 72 mg per day. The Concerta delivery system was formulated to release the MPH in a manner that re-creates the benefit of the previous regimen of 20 mg 3 times per day of immediate-release, short-acting MPH. The outer coat of the capsule is an immediate-release formulation; the paste inside provides the long-acting formulation. The 18-mg capsule, for example, is comprised of 4 mg of immediate-release as the outer coat and 14 mg of long-acting ingredient inside the capsule. A 72-mg dose of Concerta can be achieved by prescribing 4 of the 18-mg capsules per day, 2 of the 36-mg capsules, or an 18-mg capsule plus one 54-mg capsule. When taking 72 mg, the individual receives 16 mg of immediate-release formulation and 56 mg of the long-acting formulation, which is metered throughout the day in an ascending dosing manner.

Here is an effective approach to initiate Concerta in a young individual:

1. Start the regimen on a Saturday with one 18-mg capsule. While typically 18 mg is too small a dose to be effective, occasionally a child will respond.
2. If an 18-mg dose is ineffective, the individual should take two 18-mg capsules on Sunday.
3. If 36 mg are ineffective and no side effects have been noted, the individual should take three 18-mg capsules before school on Monday. To avoid questions at school, the parent can tell the teacher, "We are trying a new approach for our child and we'd like to hear back from you how our child did in school today." If the teacher reports success, then the parent knows the effective dose is 54 mg.

4. If 54 mg fail on the first day, the same dose should be given a second day. If it fails again and no side effects are noted, the dosage can be increased to four 18-mg (72 mg) capsules. If 72 mg do not prove effective, then it may be time to rethink either the diagnosis or the treatment approach. If review confirms the diagnosis, then a trial should be considered of an AMP/dAMP product.

In 2001, Adderall XR (AMP/dAMP) was FDA approved for once-daily dosing. Adderall is a mixed salt formulation, that is, it has both the levo- and dextro-rotational components of the AMPs. This medication comes as a capsule with the inner active ingredient formulated as coated beads with differing thicknesses of insulation, so that 50% of the bead formulation is released within 45 to 90 minutes, and the other 50% is released 4 hours later.

The duration of effectiveness varies from child to child. As the dose is increased, the length of effective duration is extended as well. The medication will provide 12-hour benefit when dosed appropriately. If the individual is given 10 mg of Adderall XR, he or she is receiving 5 mg initially and another 5 mg 4 hours later. If the individual needs 10 mg of AMP/dAMP in the morning and another 10 mg at noon, then the individual should be dosed with 20 mg Adderall XR (Table 1).

Table 1. Comparable Doses of Concerta and Adderall XR

Concerta (methylphenidate)	Adderall XR (amphetamine/ dextroamphetamine)
18 mg	10 mg
36/54 mg	20 mg
72 mg	30 mg

With Ritalin LA (MPH) and Adderall XR, 50% of the medication is released initially and then 4 hours later, the other 50% is released. The dextro-isomer Focalin XR (MPH) is a capsule containing coated beads, providing 8 hours of benefit. It is the stereoisomer of Ritalin LA, and its progenitor is the immediate-release, short-acting Focalin, which is the dextro-isomer of the immediate-release, short-acting Ritalin. Focalin has shown itself to be smooth for onset and offset and to give 4 hours of benefit. Immediate-release, short-acting Focalin has been shown to be a good adjunct to use in combination with the 8-hour Focalin XR or the 12-hour Concerta. When Concerta is given in the morning, its effects will decline by 6 PM. For the student who still has homework to do during the evening, adding a short-acting agent such as Focalin offers good benefit. A child taking 72 mg of Concerta receives the equivalent of 20 mg of MPH dosed 3 times per day; the appropriate Focalin dose is 10 mg, equivalent to 20 mg of MPH.

In a meta-analysis of 141 individuals (*J Am Acad Child Adolesc Psychiatry* 35(10): 1304–1313, 1996), Greenhill and colleagues established the following response rates to psychostimulants:

- 26% responded better to MPH
- 35% had a better response to the mixed AMP/dAMP salts
- 40% of the individuals responded equally well to either MPH or the mixed AMP/dAMP salts

Clinical experience shows MPH to be gentler in side effect profile than the amphetamines. Individuals who do not respond to MPH can be switched to the mixed AMP/dAMP salts. For those individuals who cannot tolerate a psychostimulant or for whom a psychostimulant is not indicated, one of the non-psychostimulants can be prescribed.

In July of 2007, the FDA approved Vyvanse (lisdexamfetamine) as an ADHD treatment approach for children ages 6 to 12. Vyvanse is a prodrug, meaning it is inactive until activated in the intestinal tract. Lysine is added to the active dexamphetamine. In the intestinal tract, the lysine is cleaved, leaving the active dexamphetamine component to provide the ADHD benefit. In June of 2008, the FDA approved Vyvanse for the treatment of ADHD in adult individuals. The studies showed Vyvanse to provide smooth benefit all day until 6pm. It demonstrated benefit with fewer side effects than its predecessors Adderall/Adderall XR. Because it is a prodrug, it also demonstrated a safer abuse profile as the contents cannot be taken intranasally or intravenously to achieve a "high."

The Transdermal MPH Delivery System

In 2006, the FDA approved Shire Pharmaceutical's ADHD medication Daytrana, the active ingredient of which is also MPH. What makes Daytrana unique is its delivery system, the transdermal patch. Absorption through the skin avoids both swallowing and the first-pass effect. This means that the active ingredient is absorbed directly into the bloodstream, avoiding breakdown in the gastrointestinal tract and liver. The patch is available in 10-mg, 15-mg, 20-mg, and 30-mg dosing strengths. Per the package insert, the patch is applied at approximately 7 AM and is removed at 4 PM. Many clinicians recommend that the individual keep the patch in place until 2 hours before bedtime. This off-label approach provides longer benefit for the individual's ADHD than the traditional 9-hour approach.

The Non-swallowing Child

Some children have difficulty swallowing pills and capsules. For these youngsters several medications are available to circumvent this difficulty. If a child prescribed MPH has difficulty swallowing, the Metadate and Ritalin LA capsules can be opened and their contents sprinkled onto food. For children needing an AMP/dAMP, AdderallXR capsules can also be opened and sprinkled on food. The Daytrana transdermal patch also offers a treatment approach that avoids the issue of swallowing altogether.

Non-psychostimulant Treatment Approaches for ADHD

Alternatives are available for individuals who do not respond well to the psychostimulants, who cannot tolerate them because of side effects, or who are not good candidates for these medications. Because of the potential impact on work or sports endeavors due to a positive urine drug screen resulting from psychostimulant use, many individuals are better candidates for non-psychostimulant treatment. Currently, Strattera (atomoxetine) is the only FDA approved non-psychostimulant medication for treating ADHD in children and adults, although other medications in this class are used in treating ADHD. The non-psychostimulant options include the tricyclic antidepressants (imipramine or desipramine), the SSRIs [Celexa (citalopram), Lexapro (escitalopram), Luvox (fluvoxamine), Paxil (paroxetine), Prozac (fluoxetine), and Zoloft (sertraline)], Provigil (modafinil), and Wellbutrin (bupropion) SR/XL (Box 3).

In the selection of a non-psychostimulant for treating an individual, issues arise related to adherence to the daily dosing. Missing a daily dose of imipramine can lead to withdrawal symptoms, including yet not limited to a withdrawal seizure. If it is to be discontinued, it is to be tapered by approximately 25% per week. Hence if the individual is taking 100 mg by mouth each day, the first week of taper will be 75 mg by mouth daily. The next week the dose is dropped to 50 mg by mouth per day for the week. Then it is tapered to 25 mg by mouth each day for a week. Then it can be discontinued at the 4th week. (Although

Box 3. Prescribing for ADHD

Whether on label or off-label, the nonpsychostimulant medications offer an advantage over psychostimulants in that they are not category II controlled substances. Prescriptions for non-psychostimulant medications can be called in to the pharmacy and refills can be written onto the prescriptions. As controlled substances under the jurisdiction of the Drug Enforcement Agency (DEA), psychostimulants can only be prescribed for 1 month at a time, with no telephone renewals allowed. In some states, prescribing psychostimulants must be done on triplicate prescription forms. Many states also require psychostimulant prescriptions to be filled within a specified period of time relative to the date the prescription was written. In Illinois, for example, prescriptions for psychostimulants must be filled within 7 days from the date of the prescription. As of December 19, 2007, the DEA implemented a new rule allowing clinicians to write sequential prescriptions allowing for 90 days/3 months of psychostimulant medication. Under this new rule, the practitioner must provide written instructions on each prescription indicating to the pharmacy the earliest date on which the prescription may be filled. The clinician must still exercise good medical judgment with regard to how often the individual should be seen, and whether or not the given individual is appropriate for the 90 day/3 month sequence of written prescriptions.

not precisely a 25% reduction each week, most practitioners will perform the taper by using 25-mg tablets, allowing the individual to taper by 25 mg every 1 to 2 weeks.) Imipramine also requires a steady serum level and thus takes time to build in the system. The serum level must be checked periodically to be sure the individual's dosing is not at a toxic level.

The medication atomoxetine also requires daily dosing to prove effective. For greatest benefit, the medication is titrated upward to 1.8 mg/kg per day. It is initiated for 4 days at 18 mg by mouth, then increased to 25 mg or 40 mg for 1 to 2 weeks; finally, it is titrated upward to 60 mg for 2 weeks if clinically indicated.

While most clinicians tend to top the dosage out at 80 mg per day, a 120-pound child or adolescent could theoretically be dosed to 98 to 100 mg based on the calculation of 1.8 mg/kg per day. Effectiveness is typically seen after 3 to 4 weeks of regular daily dosing. If the individual misses doses along the way, the true benefit is potentially disrupted. Atomoxetine requires some patience and dedication to daily dosing. For many individuals, its effectiveness is worth the dedication and the wait. Because it is metabolized by the cytochrome P_{450} system via $2D_6$, the clinician should be mindful of possible med-med interactions.

Provigil (modafinil) offers another non-psychostimulant approach to treating ADHD. Modafinil is FDA approved for treating excessive daytime sleepiness secondary to obstructive sleep apnea/hypopnea syndrome, narcolepsy, and shift work sleep disorder (see Chapter 10). It has been used off-label for several years for treating ADHD, primarily of the inattentive type, in adolescents and adults. One advantage of modafinil is that it provides the stimulant-like phenomenon of working when the individual takes it, not working when he or she doesn't and working immediately on being reintroduced. Unlike most other non-psychostimulants, which require time to build a serum level, modafinil allows for as-needed dosing. Thus, if a child takes the medication on Monday and Tuesday, and misses the Wednesday dose, the medication will be effective again on Thursday when resumed. One disadvantage is the medication's potential to decrease the effect of steroidal contraceptives by approximately 11% to 14%, an issue to be discussed with adolescent female individuals taking a steroidal contraceptive before prescribing modafinil. The mechanism of action of modafinil, while not fully understood, occurs in the hypothalamus and works at the sleep/wake center. While the medication provides some dopamine in the extracellular space, it is not thought to be specifically dopaminergic. It does not activate the nucleus accumbens or the ventral tegmental area, as do the traditional psychostimulants. It is this mesolimbic pathway that can become an avenue for abuse. By not activating this, modafinil has minimal abuse potential.

Also used off-label in treating ADHD, particularly the inattentive type, and specifically for adolescents and adults, is bupropion. Bupropion is an antidepressant medication that offers the dual-action mechanism of blockade of the presynaptic reuptake transport pumps for both dopamine and norepinephrine. Its dopaminergic blockade is its predominant function, with "mini" blockade of norepinephrine. Like modafinil, the medication has a stimulant-like benefit for treating ADHD in that it works when the individual takes it, it doesn't when he or she doesn't, and it works again immediately on being reintroduced. (This is true for its ADHD treatment, yet not for its antidepressant benefit.) Bupropion gives immediate benefit for focus, concentration, and energy when used to treat ADHD. It has the added advantage of assisting adolescents and adults to discontinue the use of cigarettes (marketed under the name of Zyban).

Use of Antiepileptic Medications for ADHD. One of the important diagnostic dilemmas is deciphering whether the individual has ADHD or evolving bipolar disorder. Some researchers have posited that ADHD is the premorbid condition yet to blossom into bipolarity. Thus, practitioners have begun to use the antiepileptic medications Depakote (divalproex sodium/valproic acid), Keppra (levetiracetam), Lamictal (lamotrigine), Tegretol (carbamazepine), Topamax (topiramate), and Trileptal (oxcarbazepine) for individuals who demonstrate angry or violent outbursts, and aggression/irritability. Such usage, while effective for many youngsters/adolescents, is off-label. Only divalproex sodium/valproic acid, lamotrigine, and carbamazepine are FDA approved for treating bipolar disorder as well as seizures (Table 2). With oxcarbazepine, serum sodium levels should be tested occasionally, monitoring for hyponatremia. When prescribing topiramate, the clinician should monitor for eye pain as a possible sign of onset of increase in intraocular pressure (glaucoma) and for cognitive dulling.

Table 2. On-label Uses and Age Guidelines for Antiepileptic Medications
Abbreviation: FDA, US Food and Drug Administration.

Medication	FDA Approved Indication	FDA Approved Age Usage
Depakote (divalproex sodium/valproic acid)	Partial and absence seizures	10 years and older
Lamictal (lamotrigine)	Generalized seizures of Lennox-Gastaut syndrome	2 years and older
Tegretol (carbamazepine)	Partial seizures, generalized seizures, mixed seizure patterns (not for absence seizures)	12 years and older
Topamax (topiramate)	Partial seizures, primary generalized tonic-clonic seizures, generalized seizures of Lennox-Gastaut syndrome	2 years and older
Trileptal (oxcarbazepine)	Partial seizures	4 years and older

The effects of these medications must be closely monitored. Baseline laboratory values and an electrocardiogram should be obtained before prescribing carbamazepine and divalproex sodium/valproic acid. Carbamazepine and divalproex sodium/valproic acid should have their serum levels evaluated on a regular basis.

The Alpha₂ Agonists. Clonidine and Tenex (guanfacine) are used to help calm aggressive behavior and hyperactivity, with clonidine tending to be more sedating initially than guanfacine. The recommended dose of clonidine should not exceed 0.4 mg a day (in divided doses). It is advisable to begin very gently, with one-quarter of a 0.1-mg tablet the first night, and monitor for sedating response. Guanfacine may be initiated at 0.5 mg the first night and then titrated cautiously as needed up to 3 mg per day in divided doses. Neither medication should be stopped abruptly, as the individual may experience rebounding hypertension. Blood pressure should be monitored as either medication is initiated and for any change in dosing.

The Atypical Antipsychotics. Some practitioners are using low doses of the atypical antipsychotic medications to help calm aggression, including Abilify (aripiprazole, a dopamine partial agonist), Geodon (ziprasidone), Risperdal (risperidone), Seroquel (quetiapine), and Zyprexa (olanzapine). Aripiprazole is initiated at 1 to 2mg per day and may be increased to 3 to 5mg as indicated. Ziprasidone is initiated at 20 mg. Risperidone is initiated at 0.25 mg at bedtime and then increased to twice-a-day dosing (3 times a day in some children), not to exceed 3 mg a day for the child or adolescent with ADHD. Quetiapine is dosed at 25 mg in the evening and may be titrated to 2 to 3 times a day dosing; daytime doses may calm hyperactivity and aggressiveness and larger nighttime doses may facilitate better nighttime sleep. Olanzapine is initiated at 2.5 mg and may be increased to twice a day dosing or 5 mg at bedtime.

These atypical antipsychotic medications have several potentially serious side effects, so individuals and their parents should be clearly warned about the risk of akathisia, dystonic reaction, metabolic syndrome, neuroleptic malignant syndrome, parkinson-like tremor, and tardive dyskinesia, among others. Quetiapine, ziprasidone, and aripiprazole are least likely to produce weight gain.

Recent FDA recommendations due to the potential for metabolic syndrome are to periodically assess individuals taking atypical antipsychotic medications for disruption in glucose metabolism (diabetes mellitus), disturbance in cholesterol levels (hypercholesterolemia), and elevations of triglycerides (hypertriglyceri-demia) (see Chapter 3).

A SUMMARY OF PHARMACOLOGIC APPROACHES TO ADHD

Psychostimulants
- Adderall/Adderall XR (AMP/dAMP)
- Concerta (MPH)
- Dexedrine (AMP)
- Desoxyn (methamphetamine)
- Focalin/Focalin XR (MPH)
- Metadate/Metadate CD (MPH)
- Methylin/Methylin ER (MPH)
- Ritalin/Ritalin LA (MPH)
- Vyvanse (lisdexamfetamine) (AMP "pro-drug")

Tricyclic Antidepressants
- Norpramin (desipramine)
- Pamelor (nortriptyline)
- Tofranil (imipramine)

Alpha$_2$ Adrenoreceptor Agonists
- Catapres (clonidine)
- Tenex (guanfacine)

Serotonin Selective Reuptake Inhibitors
- Celexa (citalopram)
- Lexapro (escitalopram)
- Luvox (fluvoxamine)
- Paxil (paroxetine)
- Prozac (fluoxetine)
- Zoloft (sertraline)

Anti-seizure Medications
- Depakote (divalproex sodium/valproic acid)
- Lamictal (lamotrigine)
- Tegretol (carbamazepine)
- Trileptal (oxcarbazepine)

Antipsychotic Medications
- Abilify (aripiprazole)
- Geodon (ziprasidone)
- Risperdal (risperidone)
- Seroquel (quetiapine)
- Zyprexa (olanzapine)

Aminoketone Antidepressant
- Wellbutrin SR/XL (bupropion)

Non-traditional Awake-Promoting Stimulant
- Provigil (modafinil)

Specific Norepinephrine Reuptake Inhibitor
- Strattera (atomoxetine)

The Risks, Side Effects, and Benefits of the Medications Used to Treat ADHD

Psychostimulants may be intermittently dosed (Goldman's Rule of Psycho-stimulants: "they work when you take them, they don't when you don't, and they work again immediately upon being re-introduced").
   Risks/Side Effects
       ❑ Monitor for abuse.
       ❑ Monitor for agitation/activation, appetite suppression, headache, motor tics, nausea, tachycardia, and thought disorganization.
       ❑ Monitor for weight loss.
   Benefits
       ❑ Available as short-acting and long-acting medications.
       ❑ Immediate onset of benefit without need to build level in serum.
       ❑ May be used on an as-needed basis as opposed to steady daily dosing.

Tricyclic antidepressants should be dosed daily without abrupt discontinuation that may cause withdrawal seizures.
   Risks/Side Effects
       ❑ Monitor for dry mouth, blurry vision, urinary retention, constipation, and slowing of cardiac conduction.
       ❑ Monitor for suicidal ideations.

- ❑ Obtain periodic serum levels to assess for therapeutic range and avoid toxicity.
- ❑ Obtain pre-initiation electrocardiogram as the medication may slow electrical conduction through the heart muscle.

Benefits
- ❑ Calm anxiety and improve mood.
- ❑ May calm impulsivity and hyperactivity.
- ❑ May improve focus and concentration.

Alpha$_2$ adrenoreceptor agonists should be dosed daily.

Risks/Side Effects
- ❑ May cause decreased mood.
- ❑ May lower blood pressure; initially monitor blood pressure before each dose and 1 to 2 hours after each dose.
- ❑ Hold dose for blood pressure reading ≤90/60 mm Hg.
- ❑ Do not discontinue abruptly, as rebounding hypertension may result.

Benefit
- ❑ Calm aggressive acting out and hyperactivity.

Serotonin selective reuptake inhibitors should be dosed daily.

Risks/Side Effects
- ❑ Monitor for agitation, akathisia, dyskinesia, headache, hyponatremia, insomnia, jitteriness, and nausea.
- ❑ Monitor for suicidal ideations.

Benefits
- ❑ Calm anxiety.
- ❑ Improve mood.
- ❑ Improve executive function.

Major mood stabilizers are used for aggressive acting out.

Risks/Side Effects
- ❑ Monitor blood levels regularly to avoid toxicity.
- ❑ Monitor for disturbance in liver function, pancreatic function, red cell count, reticulocyte count, and white cell count.
- ❑ Discontinue use if a rash occurs.
- ❑ Dosing is every day and must not stop abruptly.

Benefits
- ❑ Calm aggressive behavior.
- ❑ Improve mood.
- ❑ Stabilize mood.

Antipsychotic medications are used off-label for ADHD to treat aggressive acting out and for thought disorganization.

Risks/Side Effects

❑ Monitor for akathisia, dystonic reaction, neuroleptic malignant syndrome, parkinsonian tremor, and tardive dyskinesia.

❑ Monitor for disruption of glucose/insulin metabolism.

❑ Monitor for increased cholesterol levels (hypercholesterolemia).

❑ Monitor for increased triglyceride levels (hypertriglyceridemia).

Benefits

❑ Calm aggressive behavior.

❑ Calm tics.

❑ Improve mood.

❑ Stabilize mood.

Aminoketone antidepressant is used off-label in individuals with ADHD.

Risks/Side Effects

❑ Monitor for agitation, constipation, headache, seizures, and weight loss.

❑ Monitor for suicidal ideations.

Benefits

❑ Improve mood.

❑ Improve focus and concentration.

❑ May improve conduct disorder.

Non-traditional wake-promoting stimulant medication is used off-label in ADHD for improving energy, focus, and concentration.

Risks/Side Effects

❑ If individual is taking a steroidal contraceptive by implant, injection, pill, or transdermal patch, agent may potentially decrease the contraceptive potency by 11% to 14%.

Benefits

❑ As a non-traditional psychostimulant, it is categorized by the DEA as a category IV controlled substance and has none of the negative potential of psychostimulants.

❑ Effective for inattentive-type ADHD.

❑ Minimal abuse potential.

❑ May be used on an as-needed basis as opposed to steady daily dosing.

Specific norepinephrine reuptake inhibitor is used off-label for improving focus and concentration. It must be taken every day for 3 to 6 weeks to achieve effectiveness.

Risks/Side Effects

❑ Monitor for blood pressure elevation, nausea, reflex tachycardia, and vomiting.

❑ Monitor for liver dysfunction.

❑ Monitor for suicidal ideations.

Benefits

❑ As a nonpsychostimulant, it is not a controlled substance and has none of the negative potential of psychostimulants.

❑ Minimal abuse potential

THE 10 GUIDELINES FOR ASSESSING AND TREATING ADHD

1. Evaluate the individual and obtain a complete family history.
2. Formulate the differential diagnoses.
3. Develop a treatment plan with appropriate options.
4. Discuss risks/side effects/benefits of approaches and medications with the individual and his or her parents.
5. Formulate a treatment plan with the individual and parents with which they are comfortable.
6. Explain to the parents and individual there are no guarantees, only options based in reasonable recent scientific and clinical data.
7. Obtain informed consent for initiation of the plan.
8. Perform follow-up assessments with the flexibility to redefine the diagnosis/diagnoses as necessary.
9. Noncompliance to medication regimens can and does occur and can present as if the medication is ineffective.
10. Listen to the individual and his or her parents and teachers for feedback.

If the medication is not proving effective, the dosing regimen may not have been raised to a therapeutic level, or as noted above, the individual may not be taking the medication as prescribed. When asked how long a man's legs should be, US President Abraham Lincoln responded, "Long enough to touch the ground." When assessing for the appropriate dose of medication, the clinician should follow the precept, "enough to give benefit without causing side effects." Ultimately, an effective therapeutic regimen is the right amount of medication taken for the right amount of time. Be aware of FDA approved dosing guidelines.

COMMONLY ASKED QUESTIONS ABOUT ADHD

ADHD has a profound impact on young individuals, their families, and friends. Following are the 11 questions most commonly asked by parents and individuals.

1. What is the difference between ADD and ADHD?
ADD is the previous diagnostic name for the condition that today is technically labeled as ADHD. Three types of ADHD are recognized:
a) The inattentive type: comparable to the lay term of ADD
b) The hyperactive type: hyperactivity, impulsivity, intrusivity
c) The combined type: a combination of the inattentive type and the hyperactive type

2. When and how is the diagnosis of ADHD made?
The diagnosis of ADHD is a clinical diagnosis based on criteria as set forth by the APA in its *Diagnostic and Statistical Manual of Mental Disorders, 4th Edition-TR*:
- ADHD is typically diagnosed before the age of 7 years.
- The symptoms persist for at least 6 months.
- The symptoms are observed to be more severe and to occur more consistently than is typical for children at the same developmental stage.
- The symptoms typically occur in more than 1 setting, based on home, school, and recreation.
- The symptoms typically adversely impact the functioning in 2 or more of the above settings.

Observing the child and assessing information gathered from the individual's parents and teachers form the basis of the diagnosis.

3. Is there a blood test or scan that will diagnose ADHD?
ADHD is a clinical diagnosis, made from observation and questionnaires. Research is ongoing to develop brain-scanning techniques to assess for ADHD.

According to the APA, while these scans may be useful in confirming what has already been clinically diagnosed, they are not diagnostic in and of themselves. To date, there is no blood test for ADHD.

4. What is the treatment of choice for ADHD?

The gold standard for treating ADHD is still psychostimulant medications. Many such medications are available, falling into 2 broad categories, the MPH type and the AMP/dAMP/methamphetamine type. Each of these types is available as either short-acting, immediate-release medications or long-acting, extended-release medications.

5. What is the difference among the long-acting, extended-release medications?

The primary difference among the medications is their delivery system, i.e., the mechanism whereby the active ingredient in the medication is made available to the body and the time frame over which it is made available. Older medications use a "wax matrix" system. The newer systems are based on either "coated beads" providing time release for the medication, or the Oral Release Osmotic System (OROS®) of Concerta. The OROS is unique in its ascending dosing delivery thought to militate against tachyphylaxis, which is acute tolerance to the medication. The coated bead systems (Adderall XR, Focalin XR, Metadate CD, and Ritalin LA) allow for immediate release of one-half of the active medication, followed 4 hours later by the other one-half. Daytrana is a transdermal patch delivery system, which avoids the gastrointestinal first-pass effect seen with traditional oral medications. Vyvanse is unique in that it is a prodrug and requires activation via the gastrointestinal tract.

6. How is the medication dosed?

A therapeutic trial of medication is to give the right dose for the right amount of time providing the greatest benefit without side effects. With a medication such as Concerta, the dose may be titrated upward to 72 mg if clinically indicated and as long as no side effects are noted. With Adderall XR, the dose may be titrated upward to 30 or 40 mg. The FDA has approved dosing by weight for MPH from 1 to 2 mg/kg per day. With AMP/dAMP/methamphetamine, the FDA approves by individual weight from 0.5 to 1 mg/kg per day. Strattera is dosed from 18mg up to 60mg per day as indicated, with 1.8mg/kg as the maximum dosing guideline.

7. What if the medication is slow in onset early in the morning?

In some individuals, long-acting, extended-release medications may take too long to kick in. Parents should be advised to try the following:

- High–fat content foods may inhibit the absorption of the medication, especially AMPs/dAMPs. Make changes in the child's diet, especially at breakfast, to offer lower-fat alternatives.
- If the medication does not take effect until after the child has left for school, try gently rousing the child about an hour before his or her alarm is set to sound and give the child the medication. Allow the child to resume sleep. By the time the child wakes again, the medication should have begun to take effect and the child will be able to participate calmly in getting ready for school.
- When all else fails, give a dose of short-acting, immediate-release medication along with the long-acting, extended-release medication.

8. Can or should my child have a "drug holiday"?

A drug holiday is defined as time away from medication. While drug holidays were popular about 15 years ago, it is now recognized that ADHD doesn't take a holiday—it is present throughout the day, evening, and night. It is also recognized that adolescents are most in need of their ADHD medication on weekends and during the summer when participation in driving, dating, and other potentially dangerous and/or risky activities increases. It is important to provide the medication during the week, as well as on weekends; during the school year, as well as during vacations. The advantage of the psychostimulant medications in this regard is that they work when taken, don't work when not taken, and provide benefit again immediately on being retaken.

9. What about abuse of the psychostimulants?

Long-acting, extended-release psychostimulant medications do not give the "buzz" that might be seen with a short-acting, immediate-release medication, and hence are less likely to bring about the abuse that might be seen with short-acting, immediate-release medications. The advantage of a medication such as Concerta is that because of its capsule structure and the paste consistency of its active ingredient, the medication is not amenable to abuse or to diversion onto the street for abuse. It cannot be crushed and snorted. The Daytrana (methylphenidate) transdermal patch minimizes abuse potential. Vyvanse (lisdexamfetamine) helps protect against abuse as it is a prodrug and is activated only in the gastrointestinal tract.

10. What about combination therapy?

The treatment of ADHD is now sophisticated in the use of multiple medications for an individual. Those individuals with aggressiveness might be best served taking a combination of either an alpha$_2$ agonist such as clonidine or guanfacine or an atypical antipsychotic such as aripiprazole or ziprasidone. If the psychostimulant medication interferes with sleep or appetite, the addition of the atypical antipsychotic will often reestablish appetite/weight gain, and when given at bedtime may facilitate sleep. If the atypical antipsychotic does not help, then mirtazapine at bedtime may do so. Before initiating mirtazapine, the clinician should ask if the individual has ever taken Benadryl (diphenhydramine) and if so, what impact it had on alertness and energy. If the individual is a "paradoxical" responder to diphenhydramine and is activated, then mirtazapine should not be prescribed as it will have a similar antihistaminergic effect.

11. Will higher dosing of the psychostimulants increase the likelihood of side effects?

When prescribing a psychostimulant the goal is to reach the therapeutic threshold and stay within the therapeutic range without surpassing it. When the dose is below the therapeutic threshold, no benefit is achieved; dosing above the therapeutic range increases the potential for side effects. Sometimes gently increasing the dose still within the therapeutic range will extend the length of benefit of the psychostimulant.

CHAPTER NINE

The Cognitive Disorders

Cognitive disorders have existed since the beginning of time. Psychiatry categorizes the etiology of cognitive disorders into 3 groups:

1. Intrapsychic conflicts – These stem from the struggle between the id, the ego, and the superego and lead to disturbance in thought and cognitive function.
2. Endogenous neurochemical dysfunction – These can be either idiopathic or physiologic.
    a. Idiopathic – Just as blood pressure idiopathically goes awry, just as glucose metabolism idiopathically goes awry, so too the neurotransmitters in the brain cease to function within their "normal" parameters with resulting disturbances in cognition, motor function, and mood. When the cause is idiopathic, no readily identifiable physiologic cause is discernible.
    b. Physiologic – In these instances, internal physical disturbances such as endocrine disturbances, infectious diseases, neurologic disorders, and organ system failure result in neurochemical sequelae.
3. Exogenous stressors –Stimuli outside the body result in endogenous neurochemical dysfunction.

Historically, these disorders were referred to as *organic mental disorders, organic brain disorders, or organic brain syndrome*. The *Diagnostic and Statistical Manual of Mental Disorders, 4th Edition-TR* classifies these disorders as *cognitive disorders, mental disorders due to a general medical condition, and substance-related disorders*. The 3 major cognitive disorders are:

- Delirium
- Dementia
- Alzheimer's disease

Delirium and dementia are separate entities. Alzheimer's disease is a type of dementia. Individuals with dementia can also experience episodes of delirium.

DELIRIUM

Delirium is not a discrete disease entity; rather it is a syndrome or a pattern of symptoms indicative of an underlying physiologic disorder. Most of the causes of delirium lie outside of the central nervous system. The presence of delirium is a bad prognostic sign. The 3-month mortality rate of individuals who have an episode of delirium is estimated to be 23% to 33% and the 1-year mortality rate may be as high as 50%.

Delirium is demonstrated as the individual shows a compromise in awareness of the surrounding environment, caused by an underlying medical condition. It is characterized by disturbances in cognition, concentration, and consciousness. The signature of delirium is the disturbance in consciousness and awareness. The onset of delirium is hallmarked by rapid development, occurring from within hours to within days of initial symptoms. Its course is one of waxing and waning consciousness throughout the course of the day. Symptoms include the rapid onset of confusion, disorientation, and global cognitive impairment. It is a medical emergency due to its high mortality rate.

Another phenomenon seen in individuals with delirium is sundowning. Sundowning manifests with the individual demonstrating a worsening confusion, disorientation, and inability to focus and concentrate later in the day and into the evening, hence its name. As the sun goes down, so too the individual's focus, orientation, and mental acuity go down.

Assessing for the Cause of Delirium

Delirium is a syndrome, not a disease. When an individual presents with delirium, the clinician should begin an immediate search for the underlying cause, which can include:

- **Central nervous system causes**
  - Brain abscesses
  - Cerebral vascular accidents (stroke)
  - Status after a seizure (post-ictal state)
  - Traumatic injuries
- **Metabolic causes**
  - Atrial fibrillation/cardiac dysrhythmias
  - Cardiac ischemia
  - Febrile illness
  - Hepatic encephalopathy

- Hypoglycemia
- Hypoxia
- Illicit substance intoxication or withdrawal
- Infection
- Medication interaction, intoxication, or withdrawal
- Toxic fumes/substances

Laboratory assessment should include the following tests:
- Arterial blood gases
- Chest x-ray
- Complete blood count
- Computed tomography scan of the head
- Electrocardiogram
- Electroencephalogram
- Magnetic resonance imaging of the head
- Toxicology screen
- Urinalysis

Neurologic assessment should pay close attention to focal signs including:
- Frontal lobe release signs (suck, snout, palmomental, rooting reflexes)
- Papilledema
- Weakness or sensory loss

Once the underlying medical cause has been determined, it should be aggressively treated, if possible. To avoid exacerbating the delirium, external stimulation should be minimized and medications with significant anticholinergic effects such as Thorazine (chlorpromazine) and Mellaril (thioridazine) avoided. If the individual's delirium is the result of withdrawal from alcohol or other substance, the clinician should initiate withdrawal protocols and intervene to avoid withdrawal seizures (see Chapter 4). Agitated individuals may be calmed with low doses of high-potency antipsychotic medications such as Haldol (haloperidol), Navane (thiothixene), Orap (pimozide), Prolixin (fluphenazine), or Stelazine (trifluoperazine), or with the atypical antipsychotic medications.

DEMENTIA

Dementia is a disease characterized by multiple impairments in cognitive function without impairment in consciousness (Table 1). Dementia may be progressive or static, permanent or reversible. The potential reversibility is related to the type of dementia and to the availability and application of effective treatment.

Table 1. Comparing Delirium and Dementia

	Delirium	Dementia
Course of condition	Waxing and waning until underlying medical cause identified and treated	Progressive (rarely, it may be static)
Designation	Syndrome, caused by underlying medical condition or other identifiable source	Disease
Hallmark disruptions	3 C's: cognition, concentration, consciousness (disturbance of consciousness)	4 A's: agnosia, amnesia, aphasia, apraxia (disturbance of cognitive function)
Identifying disturbance	Disruption in consciousness	Disruption in cognitive function
Onset	Rapid	Progressive
Reversibility of condition	Typically reversible	Typically irreversible (only 3% of dementias are reversible)
Sundowning	Common	May occur later as illness progresses

Of the many types of dementias, the most common is Alzheimer's disease, accounting for 50% to 60% of cases (see below). Other common dementias are associated with:
- Vascular disease (accounting for 15%–30% of all dementia cases)
- Endocrine disorder(s)
- Infection
- Lewy body disease
- Normal pressure hydrocephalus
- Nutritional deficiencies (typically associated with alcohol abuse)
- Parkinson's disease
- Pick's disease

Fifteen percent of Americans 65 years or older suffer from mild dementia, while 5% suffer from severe dementia. Fifteen percent of Americans 80 years and older suffer from severe dementia.

As the individual with dementia begins to progress in the disease, it is common to see comorbid psychiatric conditions arise with the disruption in cognitive function:
- 20% to 30% develop hallucinations
- 30% to 40% develop delusions, primarily paranoid/persecutory
- 40% to 50% develop depression and anxiety

The Goldman Guide to Psychiatry

Normal pressure hydrocephalus is one of the treatable causes of dementia. A disorder of the drainage of cerebrospinal fluid, the condition does not progress to the point of acute increased intracranial pressure; instead it stabilizes at pressures toward the upper end of the normal range. The dilated ventricles, which may be readily seen with computed tomography scan or magnetic resonance imaging, exert pressure on the frontal lobes. A gait disorder is almost uniformly present. Less commonly, dementia that may be indistinguishable from that of Alzheimer's disease appears. The presence of a third symptom, urinary incontinence, is definitive for the diagnosis. Relief of the increased cerebrospinal fluid pressure may completely relieve the symptoms, including the dementia.

Distinguishing Between True Dementia and Confounders

Depression-Related Cognitive Impairment. Individuals suffering from depression may demonstrate disruption of cognitive functioning, so it is important to discern between depressive apathy and true dementia. While it is common for individuals with evolving dementia to become depressed, it is also possible that the cognitive disruption may be solely a result of a depressive episode; if so, successfully treating the depression will allow for return to full cognitive function. Cognitive disruption secondary to depression has been termed *pseudodementia*, as it is not a true dementia (Table 2).

Table 2. Comparison of Dementia and Pseudodementia

	Dementia	Pseudodementia
Cognitive performance on testing	Consistently poor, even with good effort	Marked variability in performance and effort
Memory	Recent memory is worse than remote memory	Recent and remote memory are equally poor
Onset	Gradual	Sudden
Past psychiatric illness(es)	None per se	Present
Individual's response to cognitive deficits	Attempts to hide	Exposes readily
Individual's response to questions	Near-miss attempts	"I don't know" response
Sundowning	Common	Rare
Vegetative signs	Not present	Present

Benign Senescent Forgetfulness (Age-Associated Memory Impairment).
Aging is not necessarily associated with any significant cognitive decline, yet minor memory problems can occur as a normal part of aging. These normal occurrences are sometimes referred to as benign senescent forgetfulness or age-associated memory impairment. They are distinguished from dementia by their minor disruption and by the fact that they do not significantly interfere with a person's social or occupational behavior.

Diagnosing Dementia

In addition to a careful physical examination, laboratory assessment, and scans, the clinician may find the Folstein Mini-Mental State Examination (MMSE) to be a quick and valuable diagnostic tool.

Understanding the Mini-Mental State Examination. The MMSE was first published in the *Journal of Psychiatric Research* in 1975. Since then it has continued to serve as a quick in-office or in-hospital method for assessing the individual's cognitive function. (A copy of the examination can be accessed at www.hartfordign.org/publications/trythis/issue03.pdf.) The MMSE is divided into 2 sections, contains 11 tasks of cognition, and requires approximately 5 to 10 minutes to administer. It has a scoring range from 0 to 30 points.

Section One relies on verbal responses and tests 3 areas for a maximum total of 21 points.

1. Orientation is assessed with questions regarding the individual's understanding of time and place (10 total points awarded).
   - Time: day, date, month, year, and season.
   - Place: location of the evaluation, the floor of the building where the evaluation is occurring, the city, the county, and the state.
2. Memory is assessed by verbally presenting 3 items to the individual (6 points).
   - The individual is asked to repeat aloud these 3 items to test registration (3 points).
   - The individual is asked to repeat them again in 5 minutes to test for immediate recall (3 points).
3. Attention is assessed either via mathematical skill testing or spelling skill (5 points).
   - The individual is asked to perform serial 7s (counting backward from 100 by intervals of 7 until the individual reaches the number 65) or

- The individual is asked to spell a 5-letter word (example: WORLD) forward and backward.

Section Two tests verbal, motor, and cognitive abilities and has 6 tasks for a maximum total of 9 points.

1. The individual's identification and verbal naming skills are assessed by being shown a pen and a watch, and asked to name each of them (2 points).
2. The individual's ability to perform verbally is assessed by being asked to repeat a tongue twister, such as "No ifs, ands, or buts" (1 point).
3. The individual's ability to follow simple sequential verbal commands is assessed by being asked, for example, to pick up a piece of paper, fold it in half, and place it onto the floor (3 points).
4. The individual's ability to follow a written command is assessed by being asked to read a written command and then follow its instructions, eg, "Please close your eyes" (1 point).
5. The individual's ability to write a sentence spontaneously is tested by being asked to write a complete sentence (1 point).
6. The individual's understanding of visual-spatial relationships is assessed by being given 2 intersecting pentagons and asked to draw the diagram created (1 point).

Interpreting the Scores from the MMSE

Traditional Scoring Values

24 to 30	Within normal limits
18 to 23	Mild-to-moderate cognitive impairment
0 to 17	Severe cognitive impairment

Goldman's Clinical Scoring Values

Many individuals with higher education have strong intellectual reserves, and the following scores are more reflective of well-educated individuals:

28 to 30	Within normal limits
24 to 28	Mild-to-moderate cognitive impairment
21 to 24	Definite moderate cognitive impairment
0 to 20	Severe cognitive impairment

Treating Dementia

Note: Before initiating any therapy, the clinician should obtain informed consent from the patient, parent, or guardian (see Appendix 1).

In treating dementia and the disorders with which it is commonly associated, clinicians should avoid medications with anticholinergic side effects. For example, if an individual with dementia is depressed and tricyclic antidepressants (TCAs) are indicated, anticholinergically the safest TCAs are Norpramin (desipramine) and Pamelor (nortriptyline). Because of potential cardiac disturbances from the tricyclic antidepressants, the serotonergic antidepressants may be a safer approach.

One-third of individuals with dementia experience psychosis. The psychotic symptoms most frequently seen are:

1. Delusions, usually of a paranoid type – Individuals often falsely believe others are hiding or stealing items from them.
2. Hallucinations – Visual hallucinations are more common in the individual with dementia than auditory hallucinations.

In treating psychosis in the individual with dementia, one must keep in mind that low-potency antipsychotic medications have the potential for sedation and anticholinergic side effects that can lead to confusion. High-potency antipsychotic medications may help to avoid the sedation and anticholinergic confusion, yet one must monitor for the motor disturbances of parkinsonism, akathisia, and dystonia. Also the clinician must be vigilant for metabolic syndrome, tardive dyskinesia and neuroleptic malignant syndrome when antipsychotic medications are prescribed.

It is currently thought that the atypical antipsychotic medications of Abilify (aripiprazole), Clozaril (clozapine), Geodon (ziprasidone), Risperdal (risperidone), Seroquel (quetiapine), and Zyprexa (olanzapine) are more effective than traditional antipsychotic medications in treating both positive and negative symptoms of psychosis. It is also believed that the atypical antipsychotic medications produce fewer side effects. However, an index of suspicion must be maintained for disturbance in glucose metabolism, hypercholesterolemia, and hypertriglyceridemia when prescribing atypical antipsychotic medications, as these are components of metabolic syndrome.

ALZHEIMER'S DISEASE
Introduction
In 1906, the neuropathologist Alois Alzheimer performed an autopsy on a patient he had first begun treating 4 years earlier. He sought to understand the

condition he had witnessed in the hospital as his patient rapidly deteriorated. In 1902, this 51-year-old Caucasian woman had presented to his care in the hospital. She had developed unexplained marital jealousy. This was followed by severe memory loss, episodes of screaming, and hallucinations. The rapid cognitive decline progressed to the point the patient no longer remembered her name or that of her husband. Then came the angry outbursts. The progression of her illness led to her inability to feed herself or toilet and ultimately to her complete "shutdown" and death. What Alzheimer saw as he gazed at her post-mortem brain were odd tangles and plaque-like structures. While he was not sure what actually caused this woman's death, he was sure that these neurofibrillary tangles and neuritic plaques caused the deterioration of her cognitive function. He presented his findings to his colleagues in the new field of neuroscience in a paper in 1907 titled "An Intriguing Disease of the Cerebral Cortex."

A century later, research has shown that the neurofibrillary tangles and neuritic plaques serve as roadblocks to the neuronal communication highway within the brain, thus disrupting the transmission of the signals of cognition. This causes the disruption of memory and visual-spatial functioning. While the tangles are thought to be a natural part of aging, having been found in the brains of individuals who never manifest any signs or symptoms of Alzheimer's disease, their formation is still a mystery. The neurofibrillary tangles are found within the neurons, while the neuritic (senile) plaques are found outside the neurons. The amyloid protein occurs naturally and through the aging process a piece becomes "clipped off." This "clipped off" piece, the beta amyloid, accumulates as deposits in the brain tissue. Another occurrence in the presence of Alzheimer's disease, or perhaps the precursor for it, is the degeneration of neurons in the nucleus basalis of Meynert where the neurotransmitter acetylcholine is manufactured. Early discoveries in neurology demonstrated that chemicals and medications that adversely impact the production and availability of acetylcholine could create a temporary memory loss. Hence, researchers have theorized that the loss of acetylcholine found in individuals diagnosed with Alzheimer's disease has an adverse impact on brain function. This current theory has led to the use of the cholinesterase (the enzyme that breaks down acetylcholine) inhibitors to slow the progress of Alzheimer's disease.

The 2 most common behavioral changes seen in individuals with dementia of the Alzheimer's type are apathy (most commonly, not interacting with others or not engaging) and agitation (occurring in 75% of Alzheimer's patients). The individual may become agitated because of environmental changes (or physical illnesses), become physically aggressive, become spontaneously reactive or impulsive, and become verbally abusive.

As Alzheimer's disease progresses, a panorama of symptoms may appear including:

- Agitation
- Anxiety
- Apathy
- Depression
- Problems with verbal communication
- Psychosis
- Sleep disturbance
- Sundowning
- Wandering

Pharmacotherapy for Alzheimer's disease

As the population of the United States ages, there is a need for greater variety of treatment approaches for the debilitating and life-threatening condition of Alzheimer's disease. This disease steals from individuals their ability to process new information and code it into memory. Not only is recent memory lost, all memory is eventually eroded as cognitive functioning declines to a completely regressive, then albeit vegetative, state, ultimately leading to death.

The first medication to be approved to treat Alzheimer's disease was Cognex (tacrine) approved by the FDA for use in the United States in 1993. Tacrine was followed by Aricept (donepezil) in 1997, quickly followed by Exelon (rivastigmine) in 2000 and Razadyne (galantamine) in 2001. The advent of these cholinesterase inhibitors to treat mild-to-moderate Alzheimer's disease was a major breakthrough in the attempt to slow the degenerative process. These medications prevent the destruction of acetylcholine by inhibiting the enzyme cholinesterase.

In 2003, Namenda (memantine), a medication that had been used in Europe for over 20 years to treat organic brain syndrome and other neurologic insults to cognitive function, was approved in the United States to treat moderate-to-severe Alzheimer's disease.

Acetylcholine and Cognition

Theory and research suggest that the part of the central nervous system which controls cognitive function is modulated and activated through neurons stimulated by acetylcholine. This cholinergic system plays a key role in learning and memory. Just as monoamine oxidase disassembles the monoamine neurotransmitters of serotonin, norepinephrine, and dopamine, so too acetylcholinesterase is the enzyme that disassembles acetylcholine. The degradation of the cholinergic system by neurofibrillary tangles and neuritic plaques is made worse with the continuing chemical degradation of acetylcholine effected by acetylcholinesterase. By blocking this enzyme, acetylcholine is allowed greater availability in the synapse enhancing cognitive function.

Memantine is not a cholinesterase inhibitor. It is an uncompetitive, voltage-dependent antagonist of the N-methyl-D-aspartate (NMDA) receptor. This receptor, which is a glutamate receptor subtype, is noted to play an important role in the functions of learning and memory. Glutamate is the activating neurotransmitter and gamma-amino-butyric acid is the inhibitory neurotransmitter. Currently, researchers believe that if the glutamate activation of the NMDA receptor becomes chronic, losing appropriate regulation, neuronal damage and death of the NMDA receptor occurs, adversely impacting learning and memory. Memantine has low-to-moderate affinity (hence minimal side effects) and rapid blocking/unblocking kinetics. It is voltage-dependent because it stays in the ion channel until a full action potential is reached. It does not respond to chronic depolarization. In addition, memantine does not compete with glutamate for the binding site. Memantine is a substitute for the magnesium ion. Magnesium serves to block the gated ion channel until a true depolarization signal occurs. The magnesium leaves the channel for an appropriate amount of calcium to flow in, and then the magnesium re-gates the channel. The chronic depolarization signal causes the magnesium to leave the channel and to not return, allowing for the unfettered influx of calcium. Memantine becomes the molecular substitute for the magnesium, moving into the ion channel and selectively gating the influx of calcium ions so the neuron is protected from the neurotoxicity of the over-influx of unregulated calcium (Box).

The cholinesterase inhibitors are approved by the US Food and Drug Administration (FDA) for treatment of mild-to-moderate Alzheimer's disease. Aricept (donepezil) is the only medication FDA approved for mild to severe Alzheimer's disease, and memantine is FDA approved for treating moderate-to-severe Alzheimer's disease. The current recommended treatment approach is the combination of a cholinesterase inhibitor plus memantine, thereby addressing multiple underlying pathologies of Alzheimer's disease.

Importance of the NMDA Receptor

Researchers believe that aside from the neurofibrillary tangles and neuritic (senile) plaques that are associated with Alzheimer's disease, disruption of the NMDA channels occurs as part of the disease process when magnesium no longer remains in place in its gated ion channel. During appropriate depolarization of the NMDA receptor, magnesium leaves the gated ion channel. On repolarization, magnesium returns to close the gate and thus stem the influx of calcium. In individuals with Alzheimer's disease, the electrical process goes awry, resulting in a chronic state of depolarization.

Memantine replaces the magnesium ion in the channel. It is a smart ion, recognizing true depolarization and not being fooled by the constant low-level electrical current that is chronic depolarization. As a result, memantine knows when to stay in the channel and when to leave it, in response to the true electrical activation of the neuron secondary to excitation caused by learning, memory, and signals of cognition.

CHAPTER TEN

Issues of Excessive Daytime Sleepiness and Fatigue

Sleep assessment is a component of the physical examination and the mental status examination. Individuals are referred to sleep labs for assessment of obstructive sleep apnea (OSA)/hypopnea syndrome (HS), narcolepsy, and other sleep disturbances. While the most common complaint presenting to the general practice physician is chest pain, the second most common complaint is, "Doc, I'm tired." The key to treating the second complaint is determining whether the individual is suffering from excessive daytime sleepiness (EDS) or excessive fatigue; these are 2 separate entities. EDS may result in the individual falling asleep in inappropriate locations and at inappropriate times. Excessive sleepiness may resolve with an adequate amount of sleep. Fatigue, on the other hand, is a condition marked by sustained exhaustion that lessens the individual's physical and mental capabilities. Rest neither fully nor consistently relieves the tiredness related to fatigue.

EXCESSIVE DAYTIME SLEEPINESS

The clinical signs of EDS are:

- Disturbances in cognition
  - Disruption in decision-making skills
  - Impairment in memory
  - Reduced vigilance
  - Slowing of information processing
  - Slowing of reaction time
- Disturbances in mood
  - Apathy
  - Irritability
  - Mood lability
- Hypnagogic hallucinations
  - Hallucinatory episodes just before sleep
- Interruptions in attention level

- Microsleep episodes
  - Falling asleep for short periods of time, even for only a few seconds

The "Big 4" culprits in the etiology of EDS are:

1. Narcolepsy
2. OSA/HS
3. Shift work sleep disorder
4. Sleep deprivation

Narcolepsy

Narcolepsy afflicts approximately 150,000 Americans. Onset is typically seen in the teens or early 20s. Its common manifestations are cataplexy, hypnagogic hallucinations, and sleep paralysis. Cataplexy, a phenomenon thought to be a hallmark of narcolepsy, is an episode of muscle weakness that may be as slight as a weakening of the jaw muscles to a full episode of knee buckling, jaw slackening, slurred speech, and vision disruption. While the individual may collapse to the ground, his or her cognitive awareness remains intact. Hypnagogic hallucinations are dream-like thoughts that occur just at the point of drifting into sleep. Hypnapompic hallucinations are the same phenomenon at the point of the individual beginning to awaken from sleep.

Obstructive Sleep Apnea/Hypopnea Syndrome

OSA and HS are commonly associated with EDS. The prevalence of sleep apnea is 2% for women and 4% for men. If left undiagnosed and untreated, the disorder is associated with substantial morbidity and mortality. The condition begins with the loss of airway tone during sleep, causing the posterior oropharynx to collapse inward and obstruct the airway. The airway obstruction arouses the sleeper, restoring airway tone, and the cycle begins anew. This is typically hallmarked by either audible gasping or loud snoring. This cycle leads to fragmented sleep and thus EDS. The obstruction also results in hypoxia, hypercapnia, and acidosis, which can cause cardiac dysrhythmias, systemic hypertension, chronic hypercapnia, pulmonary hypertension, and cor pulmonale. Hypopnea is not the complete implosion of the posterior oropharynx as found in OSA. Instead, it is shallower breathing during sleep that compromises the intake of oxygen, leading to a decrease in the amount of oxygen taken in during sleep. The resultant oxygen desaturation leads to cardiovascular, cognitive, and mood compromise. Both OSA and HS are improved via continuous positive airway pressure delivered through a face mask connected to an oxygenation machine. The pressurized input of oxygen via the mask maintains the patency of the posterior oropharynx, preventing the collapse of the airway.

Shift Work Sleep Disorder

Disturbance in the sleep/wake cycle resulting from an individual's work schedule is termed *shift work sleep disorder*. Shift work encompasses a broad area and includes individuals who do not work a traditional 9 to 5 schedule. It includes anyone whose work schedule is not synchronized with the typically perceived day/night schedule or varies daily, weekly, or monthly. Individuals who begin work before 6 AM or end work after 6 PM meet the criteria for the disorder. Thus, parents of young children, students, and those who may work a fixed shift schedule with an occasional or regular added shift are all susceptible to shift work sleep disorder (Box).

Impact of Shift Work

- Approximately 1 in 5 members of the American workforce meet the criteria of shift work.
- Approximately 2 of 3 workers on rotating shifts complain of sleep disturbances or excessive sleepiness. Fatigue is their most common complaint.
- Two of 3 shift workers report that they fall asleep on the job at least 1 day per week.
- Night shift workers are at greatest risk for job-related injuries due to sleep deprivation.
- Typical daytime employees have a 34% rate of sick leave, while shift workers report a 63% rate of sick leave.
- Shift workers commonly report headaches and stomachaches.
- Shift workers are at increased risk of heart attack.

The body's circadian rhythm matches an individual's psychological and biological rhythms. The regulator of the circadian rhythm is located in the suprachiasmatic nucleus of the hypothalamus. This nucleus regulates the body's natural rhythms of the sleep/wake cycle, body temperature, and neurochemical and hormonal release. A balance exists between the sleep drive powered by the ventrolateral preoptic nucleus and the wake drive powered by the tuberomammillary nucleus. When work patterns are out of synchronization with the body's natural circadian rhythm mechanisms, sleep/wake cycles are disrupted and individuals find themselves being sleepy at times when alertness is required and alert at times when sleep should be occurring. This results in sleep deprivation (see below) and excessive "daytime" sleepiness corresponding to the individual's daytime, whatever time that may actually prove to be.

Individuals who work "shifting" schedules are at risk for disrupting the natural neurochemical biorhythms. In the *Diagnostic and Statistical Manual of Mental Disorders, 4th Edition-TR*, the disorder is designated as a form of circadian rhythm sleep disorder. Its symptoms include disturbances in concentration, extreme sleepiness, headaches, and insomnia.

Sleep Deprivation
Sleep deprivation is the most common cause of sleepiness in the United States. The average adult requires between 8 and 8.5 hours of uninterrupted sleep per night. Most Americans fall short of this, typically receiving 6.9 hours of sleep on weeknights and 7.5 hours on weekends. Humans are programmed for a 24-hour cycle of sleep and wakefulness. Disruptions of this circadian pattern lead to sleep deprivation. Those who are at greatest risk for this disruption are most notably airline pilots, nurses, parents, physicians, shift workers, teenagers, and truck drivers. Sequelae of sleep deprivation include:

- Difficulty managing stress
- Disturbances in concentration and focus
- Disturbances in glucose metabolism
- Disturbances in memory
- Disturbances in the immune system
- Gastrointestinal disturbances
- Irritability
- Mood lability
- Sleepiness
- Vague somatic complaints
- Visual disturbances
- Weight gain

Food is to hunger as sleep is to sleepiness—there is no substitute for a good night's sleep.

FATIGUE

From the psychiatric perspective, persistent fatigue associated with major depressive disorder is the most common presentation of clinically important fatigue (see also Chapter 1). Major depressive disorder is responsible for more than 10 million physician office visits per year, with 25% of women and 15% of men experiencing at least 1 episode in their lifetime. There is a 50% recurrence rate after a first episode and an 80% recurrence rate after the third episode. Even when antidepressant medication successfully improves mood, there may still be a residual and persistent fatigue.

THE COST OF EDS AND FATIGUE

Both EDS and fatigue have a dramatic impact on individuals' lives and in the life of society itself. Thirty-seven percent of Americans polled with regard to fatigue and sleepiness report they are so sleepy that it interferes with their daily activities at least several days a month and 16% report interference with daily activities at least several days per week. The direct cost to the US economy from excessive daytime sleepiness and fatigue is estimated to be $15.9 billion annually. It is estimated that 100,000 times a year a sober driver with no passengers in the vehicle veers off the road without any attempt to return to the road, secondary to excessive sleepiness. Such accidents account for 40,000 injuries, with 1550 deaths. These numbers do not include multiple car accidents nor do they include accidents that occur with the vehicle still on the roadway.

DIAGNOSING EDS AND FATIGUE

As sleepiness and fatigue can be symptoms of various physical disorders, a complete workup is important and typically includes:

- Cardiac screening.
- Complete blood count with platelet count and reticulocyte count
- Liver panel
- Metabolic panel
- Physical examination
- Pulmonary function testing
- Sedimentation rate

- Tests for the Epstein-Barr virus, Lyme disease, human immunodeficiency virus, hepatitis virus, carboxyhemoglobin (to rule out exposure to carbon monoxide), purified protein derivative (for tuberculosis), ferritin, and total iron-binding capacity
- Thyroid panel

In addition, 2 validated self-assessments should be completed, the Epworth Sleepiness Scale (Figure 1) and the Fatigue Severity Scale (Figure 2). These instruments provide insight into the scope of the condition as well as a quantifiable number that allows tracking the individual's progress over time.

Epworth Sleepiness Scale (ESS)

Situation	Chance of dozing (0-3)			
Sitting and reading	0	1	2	3
Watching television	0	1	2	3
Sitting inactive in a public place — for example, a theater or meeting	0	1	2	3
As a passanger in a car for an hour without a break	0	1	2	3
Lying down to read in the afternoon	0	1	2	3
Sitting and talking to someone	0	1	2	3
Sitting quietly after lunch (when you've had no alcohol)	0	1	2	3
In a car, while stopped in traffic	0	1	2	3

0 = Would never doze   2 = Moderate chance of dozing
1 = Slight chance of dozing   3 = High chance of dozing

Total Score [ ]

ESS total score ≥ 10 indicates possible excessive sleepiness or sleep disorder

SOURCE: Johns MR. A new method of measuring daytime sleepiness: The Epworth Sleepiness Scale. Sleep 14(6):540-545, 1991. Reproduced with permission.

Figure 1. The Epworth Sleepiness Scale.

If the individual's total score on the Epworth Sleepiness Scale is less than 10, it is within normal range. Individuals scoring greater than or equal to 10 are suffering from EDS, and a score greater than 16 indicates severe EDS. A mean score on the Fatigue Severity Scale greater than or equal to 4 qualifies for severe fatigue.

Fatigue Severity Scale (FSS)

During the past week I have found that	Disagree ←――――――→ Agree						
My motivation is lower when I am fatigued	1	2	3	4	5	6	7
Exercise brings on my fatigue	1	2	3	4	5	6	7
I am easily fatigued	1	2	3	4	5	6	7
Fatigue interferes with my physical functioning	1	2	3	4	5	6	7
Fatigue causes frequent problems for me	1	2	3	4	5	6	7
My fatigue prevents sustained physical functioning	1	2	3	4	5	6	7
Fatigue interferes with carrying out responsibilities	1	2	3	4	5	6	7
Fatigue is among my three most disabling symptoms	1	2	3	4	5	6	7
Fatigue interferes with work, family, or social life	1	2	3	4	5	6	7

	Total Score	
FSS mean score = total score for 9 items divided by 9	**Mean Score**	
FSS mean score ≥ 4 indicate severe fatigue	Krupp LB et al. The Fatigue Severity Scale: Application to patents with multiple sclerosis and systemic Lupus erythematosus. *Arch Neurol.* 1989; 46:1121-3.	

Figure 2. The Fatigue Severity Scale.

TREATING EDS AND FATIGUE

Note: Before initiating any therapy, the clinician should obtain informed consent from the patient, parent, or guardian (see Appendix 1).

The algorithm for treating these conditions is as follows:

- Assess for sleep patterns and initiate good sleep hygiene
- Assess for OSA/HS
- Assess for narcolepsy
- Assess for shift work sleep disorder
- Evaluate appropriateness for pharmacotherapy

When considering either OSA/HS or narcolepsy as possible causes of excessive daytime sleepiness, the clinician can make a definitive diagnosis with a sleep study. Today most moderately sized cities and most hospitals have sleep laboratories established for performing the necessary sleep studies.

Continuous positive airway pressure is the current gold standard of initial care for individuals with OSA. Continuous positive airway pressure delivered through a face mask connected to an oxygenation machine maintains the patency of the posterior oropharynx. Individuals who do not respond are candidates for adjunctive pharmacotherapy with the psychostimulants or Provigil (modafinil). Provigil (modafinil) is approved by the US Food and Drug Administration (FDA) for treating residual EDS secondary to OSA.

Psychostimulants and Provigil (Modafinil)

The traditional approach for treating EDS or fatigue secondary to OSA/HS and narcolepsy has been the psychostimulants. These are the same medications used in treating attention-deficit/hyperactivity disorder (see Chapter 8). Methylphenidate, amphetamine, and dextroamphetamine formulations are standard treatment approaches. Long-acting formulations offer the advantage of dosing before work for an 8-hour workday. The traditional psychostimulants provide the benefit of alerting the individual and enhancing focus and concentration. The downside is that traditional psychostimulants have the potential to disturb sleep architecture, suppress appetite, exacerbate underlying anxiety disorders, increase heart rate, elevate blood pressure, and lead to abuse and dependence. The traditional psychostimulants offer 4 hours of benefit with short-acting, immediate-release formulae and 8 to 12 hours of benefit when given as the long-acting, slow-release formulations.

Provigil (modafinil) is a nontraditional alerting medication that is specifically FDA approved for treating EDS and fatigue associated with narcolepsy, OSA/HS, and shift work sleep disorder. Like the psychostimulants, modafinil works when the individual takes it, doesn't work when he or she doesn't, and works again immediately on resumption. Individuals do not feel a buzz or a jolt of energy when they take the medication; instead they notice at the end of the day that they have been awake and alert throughout the day and able to complete tasks competently. According to the package insert for modafinil, 200 to 400 mg a day is the FDA approved dosing amount. As some individuals see benefit from just 100 mg per day, it is advisable to start modafinil at 100 mg by mouth in the morning for several days, at which time the individual can reassess symptoms. If the fatigue or EDS persists, the individual can try taking 100 mg in the morning and 100 mg in the afternoon; ultimately, some may need 200 mg twice a day. For most individuals, the 15-hour half-life allows for once-daily dosing. If the medication is dosed 2 times a day, a steady state serum level is achieved. Because the mechanism of action of modafinil is not specifically dopaminergic and the medication focuses on the sleep/wake center in the hypothalamus, it typically does not adversely impact sleep. While this medication enhances alertness, it does not disrupt sleep architecture. Because it focuses on the hypothalamus and does not cause dopamine to be activated from the ventral tegmental area to the nucleus accumbens as do the traditional stimulants, modafinil has minimal abuse potential.

A few individuals may need off-label dosing of 400 mg or more twice a day to gain benefit. The key with any medication is to provide benefit without side effects. When prescribing any medication outside the FDA approved usage guidelines, the clinician should obtain informed consent from the patient (or parents/guardian) who has been advised that the dosing regimen is outside the FDA approved parameters (see Appendix 1).

For medications inducing sleep, review the sleep algorithm found in Appendix 2.

CHAPTER ELEVEN

The Somatic Triad in Psychiatry

The clinician may encounter 3 conditions in which individuals either create their signs and symptoms to fulfill a conscious agenda or experience these signs and symptoms as an attempt to resolve an underlying unconscious conflict. Symptom formation occurs at the conscious level in 2 of these conditions—factitious disorder and malingering—and at the unconscious level for 1—somatoform disorder. What distinguishes these conditions from each other and from all other psychiatric conditions is the primary and secondary gain achieved in each condition (Box). Somatoform disorder and factitious disorder are the result of intrapsychic conflicts the individual is seeking to resolve.

SOMATOFORM DISORDER

Somatoform disorder, known eponymously as Briquet's syndrome, was named after Paul Briquet, who described this phenomenon in 1859. The individual's underlying intrapsychic conflict is not being allowed center stage in the individual's conscious mind and is relegated to the unconscious. As this intrapsychic energy persists, it presses against the unconscious defense mechanisms of denial and repression and the conscious defense mechanism of suppression. While both the unconscious and the conscious seek to keep this conflict and its problematic intrapsychic energy silent, the conflict will find a way to be heard via physical manifestation(s). The symptoms manifest physiologically, yet do not have a true underlying physiologic cause. The physical complaint eventually drives the individual to the clinician. Over time, the clinician or others involved in the individual's care discern the psychiatric cause. Five types of somatoform disorder have been delineated.

Body Dysmorphic Disorder

In body dysmorphic disorder, the individual is preoccupied with a given body part or area. This preoccupation becomes so exaggerated or distorted in the individual's mind that it may take on the qualities of a delusional disorder. This is often seen in individuals who are preoccupied with the shape of their nose (leading to rhinoplasty), their abdomen and thighs (leading to liposuction), or

Primary Versus Secondary Gain

Sigmund Freud developed the concept of psychoanalysis and with it two constructs of the mind. He developed a structural construct comprised of the id, ego, and superego and a topographical construct comprised of the conscious, preconscious, and unconscious (see Chapter 13). These 3 structural components are often found in conflict, which occurs topographically in the unconscious mind. This conflict is resolved by bringing the information from the unconscious mind into the conscious mind, a process that can prove emotionally painful. To avoid the painful experience, the individual's mind seeks to keep this conflict at the unconscious level, in its unresolved state. This process of rejecting the unconscious conflicted information is the domain of the defense mechanisms and is referred to as *resistance*. The role of the therapist is to assist the individual in "working through the resistance." When an individual maintains the resistance, he or she may benefit in 1 of 2 ways:

Primary Gain – This is the trade-off the individual makes to avoid emotional discomfort by preventing the unconscious conflict from being brought to light in the conscious mind. The avoidance of the emotional pain is the gain or benefit, which occurs at the unconscious level. The purpose of psychoanalysis is to allow the individual to work through the resistance to achieve conscious insight and hence gain mastery over the internal resistances. Gaining mastery allows the individual to resolve the unresolved intrapsychic conflict. Primary gain is the benefit from keeping the conflict unresolved and repressed thereby avoiding the painful process of gaining insight.

Secondary Gain – This is the component of benefit translated into social, physical, or financial benefit from one's illness. The underlying drive is unconscious and the benefit is external.

their physique (leading to breast augmentation or reduction). For this to become a true body dysmorphic disorder, the concern must cause the individual significant distress or be associated with impairment in the individual's personal, social, or occupational life.

Conversion Disorder

This subtype of somatoform disorder produces neurologic disturbances. It is characterized by 1 or several symptoms, with the most common being distortion of feeling (paresthesias), disturbance in 1 or several of the 5 senses, or paralysis of 1 or several limbs. The case of Anna O, a patient of Sigmund Freud and Joseph Breuer, is the classic case on which this condition is based (see Chapter 13). While the signs and symptoms in individuals with conversion disorder present as neurologically based, no medical or neurologic explanation can be found for the individual's condition.

Hypochondriasis

Individuals suffering from hypochondriasis constantly and consistently complain of vague or specific physical ills with no underlying medical or neurologic explanation. The word *hypochondriasis* comes from the medical term *hypochondrium*, meaning "below the ribs" and refers to the typical presentation of abdominal complaints. This condition usually results from the individual's unrealistic and/or inaccurate interpretation(s) of physical symptoms or sensations that cause the individual to experience a preoccupation with and fear of having or contracting a serious disease. This preoccupation and fear disrupts the individual's ability to function in social and occupational roles.

Pain Disorder

As the name indicates, the primary complaint of individuals with pain disorder is pain in 1 or more physical sites. The symptoms are associated with emotional distress and cause functional impairment, with no medical or neurologic explanation forthcoming from examination, laboratory assessment, or radiologic scans.

Somatization Disorder

Symptoms of somatization disorder present before the age of 30 years and cause the individual significant psychological distress and disruption in social and work functioning. The individual is on a constant quest for medical evaluations and interventions and has many physical complaints, none of which can be explained based on laboratory results or physical examination. In making this diagnosis, the clinician should look for the following combination of signs and symptoms:

- Pain in 4 different areas or systems of the body
- A minimum of 2 symptoms related specifically to the gastrointestinal tract
- A minimum of 1 sexual disturbance
- A minimum of 1 neurologic disturbance

While these symptoms need not occur concurrently, they must occur over the period of the condition. Once the correct diagnosis is made, the individual must be treated psychiatrically as opposed to medically, as there is no underlying physical cause for the somatic complaints.

FACTITIOUS DISORDER

Individuals with factitious disorder consciously create symptoms with the specific purpose of being in the sick role. While the production of symptoms occurs at the conscious level, the drive to produce these symptoms comes from an unconscious intrapsychic need for attention. Three types of factitious disorder with interesting nuances among them are commonly seen.

Primarily Psychological Type

These individuals falsely create the loss of a loved one to engage in factitious bereavement, feign symptoms of psychosis with false hallucinations, or complain of a disturbance in memory by feigning dementia. This form of factitious disorder has 2 interesting variants. *Pseudologia fantastica* occurs when the individual combines some factual material with incredible and colorful fantasies. *Impostorship* involves the individual assuming a role more important than his or her true-life role. Claiming to be a war hero or from an important family are examples of impostorship.

Primarily Physical Type

There are two subtypes of the physical type of factitious disorder. Both subtypes satisfy the unconscious intrapsychic conflict via elaborate and ongoing physical symptoms. Both subtypes manifest their symptoms through the conscious efforts of the individual. Subtype one, eponymously named *von Munchausen syndrome* after Baron von Munchausen, directly involves the individual. The 18th-century German baron was noted for the adventure stories he wrote of his many travels. His stories were reported as quite expansive, grandiose, and perceived as having inflated the truth. In 1951, British psychiatrist, Sir Richard Asher, gave Baron von Munchausen's name eponymously to individuals who presented with fabricated symptoms of illness. Most notable is the individual's ability to present the physical signs and symptoms so well that he or she is commonly admitted to the hospital. Once hospitalized, he or she wishes to remain in the sick role and may prove very demanding and difficult toward staff. As the clinician orders more and more tests, and as each comes back negative or within normal limits, the individual, fearing discharge from the sick role, may become verbally abusive (accusing the clinician of incompetence) or threaten litigation. These individuals will create symptoms by falsifying records, inducing self-injury, and/or contaminating laboratory samples. For example, the individual may add sugar to a urine sample to show increased glucose in the urinalysis.

Subtype two is a variation in which the individual obtains status from the sick role by proxy. The person suffering from this psychiatric disorder, known as *von Munchausen by proxy*, intentionally produces physical signs or symptoms in another individual who is under the person's care. Hence the caretaker is able to vicariously enjoy the sick role. This is typically a mother who often works in the health care field and deceives medical personnel into believing her child is ill. The mother will falsify records, contaminate laboratory samples, or even induce injury or illness in her child.

Combined Type

This is the individual who creates a combination of psychological and physical symptoms to obtain medical attention and concern.

MALINGERING

Of all the diagnoses made in medicine and psychiatry, the diagnosis of malingering is given the least often. When given, it is done with reluctance. Clinicians hesitate to give this label to an individual because it is the only diagnosis that questions the individual's veracity. In very plain terms, when clinicians give this diagnosis, they are calling the individual a prevaricator or liar. Once this diagnosis is given, the clinician is at risk for being sued for defaming the individual. Since truth is an absolute defense against a lawsuit for libel or slander, the clinician must be absolutely certain of this diagnosis before making it. Malingerers create their signs and symptoms at a conscious level for conscious goals and rewards. Malingering is an example of secondary gain of a conscious nature.

- Individuals engage in malingering to be hospitalized. This may be done to secure financial compensation, as in an automobile accident in which no real injury has occurred. The malingerer can feign symptoms well enough to win a large jury award or insurance settlement. Other reasons a malingerer may seek hospitalization include evading the police, avoiding work, or obtaining free services.
- Individuals engage in malingering to avoid the consequences of criminal activity. Since psychiatric illnesses are diagnosed clinically and not by laboratory evaluation or radiologic scans, individuals often feign psychiatric symptoms to appear incompetent at the time of the commission of the offense or incompetent to stand trial, or to demonstrate diminished capacity so as to receive a lesser sentence.
- Individuals engage in malingering to avoid being drafted into the military. Individuals already in the military may feign symptoms to obtain a discharge, avoid undesirable military assignments, or avoid combat duty.
- Individuals engage in malingering to obtain Social Security disability payments, veteran's benefits, worker's compensation benefits, and other financial rewards.
- Individuals engage in malingering as inmates in correctional facilities to obtain medications (often for abuse purposes) or be transferred to a psychiatric unit for more comfort.

To summarize, somatoform disorder refers to individuals who present with medical symptoms that are not consciously created and occur due to unresolved unconscious conflict. Factitious disorder refers to individuals who consciously feign symptoms to be in the sick role for unconscious reasons. Malingering refers to individuals who consciously create symptoms of mental or physical illness for the conscious purpose of monetary gain or to avoid an unwanted consequence.

	Unconscious Symptom Formation	Conscious Symptom Formation
Unconscious Conflict	Somatoform Disorder	Factitious Disorder
No Unconscious Conflict (fulfilling a Conscious Desire)		Malingering

CHAPTER TWELVE

The Initial Interview and Evaluation

The initial psychiatric evaluation of the individual by the clinician is comprised of the history gathering portion and the Mental Status Exam (MSE). The MSE is to the psychiatrist what the physical examination is to the family practitioner; it is the process whereby the psychiatrist observes and listens to the individual. The psychiatrist observes dress, facial expressions, grooming, motor movements, and the individual's interaction with the psychiatrist. While the MSE is key to assessing the health and status of the individual's mind, social skills, and cognitive function, it is by no means the only information gathered during the interview. The traditional structure for the interview is as follows:

- Chief complaint
- History of present illness
- Past medical history
- Review of systems
- Current medications
- Past medications
- Allergies/allergies to medication
- Social history
  - Substance use/abuse
  - Sexual history
  - History of any abuse: sexual, physical, emotional
  - Legal history
  - Military history: military service, combat, type of discharge
- Family history
  - Medical
  - Psychiatric
- Past psychiatric history
- The Mental Status Exam (MSE)
- Diagnostic impressions (5 axis diagnoses – the 5 axes)
- Treatment plan

GOLDMAN'S TIME-SAVING AND INDIVIDUAL-FRIENDLY INTERVIEW TECHNIQUE

While the above sequence is widely favored by residency training programs, eliciting the information in another sequence, as outlined below, often speeds the interview process and puts the individual more at ease early in the process. Whether in the emergency department or an outpatient office, the initial interview serves 3 important purposes: (1) to gather data; (2) to help the individual begin the process of developing insight; and (3) to establish rapport with the individual. Of these, establishing rapport is of critical importance. Individuals who feel comfortable with their evaluating and treating clinician will answer questions and allow the clinician to return to ask more questions at a later time. Below is the process for obtaining information while establishing a comfortable relationship with the individual.

In this revised sequence, the clinician does not begin with the chief complaint. The individual's current psychiatric history is essentially the psychiatric chief complaint. It is important to wait to ask "What is bringing you here today?" until the very end of the interview. Asking that question at the outset of the interview often results in the individual becoming emotionally distraught, with the rest of the interview being spent putting the individual back together. Should that happen, no other information will be gathered and the MSE will be incomplete. Goldman's Time-Saving Individual-Friendly Interview is as follows:

Allergies to Medications

The interview begins with asking about medication allergies. This information is crucial so as to avoid improperly prescribing a medication to which the individual has a pre-existing allergy. The individual-friendly reasons to begin with this question are 2-fold:

1. Individuals are usually anxious about being seen by a psychiatrist or in a mental health setting. By beginning with a medical question, the clinician allows the individual to begin to feel more at ease because he or she can see the process as medical first.
2. If the individual acknowledges allergies to any psychiatric medications, it provides the clinician with early information into the individual's past psychiatric history as well as insights into the individual's diagnosis. It also opens the door for questions about past and present psychiatric history as a natural segue.

Past Medical History

Questions about the individual's past medical history are the second series of questions. These questions about any surgeries or medical illnesses reinforce the medical nature of the interview. The clinician establishes a pattern early in the interview for the individual to be conditioned to being asked questions and answering them. This allows the individual to relax into the process.

Review of Systems

A review of systems is more general than the above past medical history. The clinician may say to the individual: "I am now going to ask questions from the top of your head to the tips of your toes, and it won't even tickle" (observing the response, to see if it evokes a smile). Questions review the major physical systems of auditory, cardiovascular, dermatologic, digestive, endocrine, hematologic, muscular, neurologic, respiratory, reproductive, urogenital, and visual.

Social History

Questions related to the individual's social history provide broad-based information about the individual's life, including questions about marital status, relationship status, status of having children, where the individual lives and with whom. For children and adolescents, questions relate to school activities; for adults, to employment. Also included within the social history are questions about:

- Abuse history – It is important to ask about any past or present emotional, physical, or sexual abuse.
- Legal history – It is important to ascertain whether the individual has any outstanding legal issues. Is the individual currently on probation? If so, for what? Has the individual been cited for driving under the influence of alcohol or other substance? Has the individual ever been arrested or served time in jail or prison? Are there any pending legal charges or legal proceedings? The individual's answers can provide insight into possible substance abuse, anger-management issues, and other behavioral issues. These answers also provide perspective with regard to the individual's judgment.
- Military service – Has the individual served in the military? If so which branch? List the years of service. Did the individual experience combat? What type of discharge did the individual receive?
- Sexual history – Every individual should be asked about past and current sexual activity, including any history of sexually transmitted diseases. Sexually transmitted diseases such as syphilis and human immunodeficiency

virus can adversely impact neurologic functioning, thereby impacting mood, cognitive function, and motor function. Sexually transmitted diseases such as chlamydia, human papilloma virus (genital warts), and/or genital herpes can adversely impact the individual's self-esteem, contributing to a decline in mood. If the individual is a woman of childbearing age, pregnancy may be the underlying cause of the changes in mood and behavior. Before the clinician prescribes any medication, women of childbearing age should be assessed for pregnancy by either obtaining a urine pregnancy test or serum beta human chorionic gonadotropin test.

• Substance use – Every individual should be asked about use of alcohol, caffeine, nicotine, cocaine, hallucinogens, inhalants, intravenous use of substances, and/or marijuana. When indicated a urine drug screen is ordered.

By shifting from the medical questions to the social history, the clinician is transitioning the individual to life-related questions. So as not to lose rapport with the individual, the interview now shifts back to a medical model approach.

Current Medications

This step allows the clinician to compile a list of the medications the individual is currently taking. This includes vitamins and food supplements as well as prescription medications. If any of these medications are for psychiatric disorders, the clinician is afforded a good segue to ask the individual about past and current psychiatric history.

Past Medications

Asking the individual about past prescribed medications provides insight into what other clinicians, physicians and psychiatrists have thought of the individual's medical and psychiatric condition(s). This information may indirectly reveal if the individual was treated for a specific psychiatric condition that the individual may be hesitant to discuss. In addition, individuals are not always clear about their past diagnoses; knowing the past medications can often help the clinician assess what the prior diagnoses have been. If the individual has taken specific medications in the past, follow-up questions include:

• What was the dose?
• Were there any side effects?
• Was the medication effective?
• Do you feel that you would benefit from being on that medication again?
• What led you to discontinue the medication in the past?

- When was the last time you took the medication?
- Who prescribed the medication for you?
- Was the medication the branded medication or a generic?
- Did you or the clinician notice a difference in benefit between the branded medication and its generic counterpart?
- Do you recall the reason the medication was prescribed?

The answers not only assist the clinician in making the diagnosis, the answers also assist in devising a treatment plan that does not duplicate previous ineffective therapy.

Family History

Questions about both medical and psychiatric family history allow for a natural segue into the individual's psychiatric history. Family history is important in assessing genetic loading for physical and psychiatric illnesses. These questions focus on the individual's knowledge of illnesses of immediate family members, including time frames. Caution is advised before proceeding to the individual's past psychiatric history. It is important to be able to separate the past psychiatric history from the current psychiatric history (psychiatric chief complaint). At this point in the interview, questions move to the individual's past psychiatric history; if necessary, the clinician should ask the individual to reserve discussing the current psychiatric issue/chief complaint until after the MSE is completed.

Psychiatric History

The individual's psychiatric history consists of direct questions about past visits to a psychiatrist or other mental health clinician, hospitalizations, and treatments. These questions include:

- Have you ever been to a counselor, social worker, psychologist, or psychiatrist?
- Have you been to a medical clinician for any disturbance in behavior, mood, or thought?
- Have you ever been given a psychiatric diagnosis?
- Have you ever been in the hospital for psychiatric reasons?
- Have you ever been in a substance treatment program?
- Have you ever had electroconvulsive therapy (ECT)?
- Have you ever taken psychiatric medications?

This completes the questions and assessment leading up to the MSE. Following the MSE, the individual is asked about his or her current chief complaint.

The Mental Status Examination (MSE)

The MSE can be prefaced with a comment such as, "I am going to shift gears and ask you a set of questions I ask everybody. This is an important part of our meeting today. Some of these questions may seem very simple to you. At times I may sound like a game show host. Please bear with me." And then the clinician proceeds by asking the following questions:

1. Can you tell me your name? [Orientation to Person]
2. Can you tell me what city we are in? What county? What state? [Orientation to Place]
3. Can you tell me what month it is right now? [Orientation to Time]
4. Can you tell me what year it is? [Orientation to Time]
5. Can you tell me what day it is? The day of the week? Today's date? [Orientation to Time]
6. Can you tell me who the president of the United States is today? [Recent Memory]
7. Can you tell me who was president immediately before him or her? [Intermediate Memory]
8. And do you remember who it was immediately before that? [Longer Term Memory]
9. And how about immediately before that? [Remote Memory]
10. I am going to ask you to spell a word for me. Can you spell the word WORLD? [Cognitive Function]
11. Now can you spell that word backward? [Testing Concentration] (Note: instead of having the individual spell a word forward and backward to test concentration, some clinicians will use the testing technique of "serial 7's". In this technique the individual is told the following: "In a moment I will start you with the number 100. I will ask you to subtract 7 from that. This will leave you with a new number. Then I will want you to subtract 7 from that. Then I will want you to take that new number and subtract 7 from it, and so on and so forth until I tell you to stop." Typically the clinician will allow the individual to proceed from 100 to 65 and then stop the individual. The clinician is to chart each of the individual's answers and make no comment as to whether or not each step along the way is correct or incorrect.)
12. You know what an apple is and you know what an orange is. How are they alike? How are they similar? [Testing Abstract Thinking]

13. You know what a cat is and you know what a dog is. How are they alike? How are they similar? [Testing Abstract Thinking]

14. You know what a knife is and you know what a fork is. How are they alike? How are they similar? [Testing Abstract Thinking]

15. You know what a fly is and you know what a tree is. How are they alike? How are they similar? [Testing Abstract Thinking]

16. I am going to give you 3 words and ask you to tuck them away into your memory; I will come back to them in about 5 minutes and ask you to recall them. They are "blue, chair, friendship." Then ask the individual to repeat them and record that the individual heard the words and properly repeated them, thus showing intact registration. Proceed with the MSE, keeping track of the time, and ask the individual to recall the 3 words 5 minutes later. Record the individual's response and the order in which the words are recalled. [Testing immediate recall]

17. Now I am going to ask you the Big 6, then the Big 3, and then 1 main question, the big one, okay?

What follows are questions about the 6 neurovegetative functioning inventory indices to assess the criteria for depressive disorder, bipolar disorder, anxiety disorder, and/or thought disorder (see Chapter 1). The mnemonic **SAMCEL(S)** highlights the 6 areas: **S**leep, **A**ppetite, **M**emory, **C**oncentration, **E**nergy, and **L**ibido (the 6 neurovegetative functioning inventory indices), plus **S**uicidal/Homicidal ideations. While many clinicians prefer to assess the neurovegetative functioning inventory indices during the history of present illness section, the MSE provides a logical and meaningful place to assess and record these key questions. These indices involve the following questions:

S: How are you sleeping? Are you having any difficulties falling asleep (sleep initiation), staying asleep (sleep maintenance), or awakening from sleep (timely morning arousal from sleep)?

A: Any changes in your eating habits? Are you gaining or losing weight? Is your appetite at its usual level? Is it decreased? Is it increased?

M: Any changes in your ability to remember?

C: Any difficulties with concentration, staying on target, staying on task, or staying on track?

E: How is your "get up and go"? Any problems performing tasks during the day?

L: How is your libido? Freud narrowly defined libido as interest in sexual activity. How is that for you? Do you find that your thoughts have increased or decreased? Do you feel your interest in sexual activities is where it should be? Are you concerned about it?

S: Any thoughts of wanting to hurt yourself or someone else, or of killing yourself or someone else (suicidal ideations and/or homicidal ideations)? Any thoughts of wanting to die?

When the individual identifies changes in any of the neurovegetative functioning inventory indices, ask when the change began and how long it has persisted. Using SAMCEL(S) allows the clinician to assess for mood disorders, anxiety disorders, thought disorders, ADHD, sleep disorders, as well as enhancing the index of suspicion for medical illnesses.

While the final "S" of SAMCEL(S) includes suicidal ideations and homicidal ideations, the "Big 3" revisits these issues and expands on them. The Big 3, questions that must be asked in every interview and at every session, are all about safety—the individual's and that of those around him or her. In any interview or session, if the clinician can only ask 3 questions, they would be:

1. Are you having hallucinations, auditory, visual, or tactile?
2. Have you thought about hurting or killing someone?
3. Have you thought about hurting or killing yourself?

It is essential to ask these 3 questions and record the individual's responses in the medical chart. If the individual responds in the affirmative to any of these 3 questions, additional questioning should follow to assess the level of risk to the individual and others.

In the case of hallucinations, it is important to determine if the individual is experiencing auditory hallucinations of a command type. If the individual is hearing voices, are the voices telling the individual to hurt himself or herself or to hurt someone else?

In the case of homicidal ideations, is the individual seriously intent on hurting or killing someone else? Can or will the individual identify a specific person as the potential victim?

In the case of suicide, follow-up questions include:

- Are you having any thoughts of wanting to hurt yourself?
- Are you having any thoughts of dying?
- Are you having any thoughts of wanting to kill yourself?
- When was the last time you had these thoughts?
- Have you ever acted on these thoughts before? If so, please describe what you did.
- Do you have a plan now? If so, what is it?
- Do you currently have the intent to act on the plan? Do you have the tools necessary to complete your plan?

The purpose of these additional questions is to determine where the individual's suicidal ideations lie on a passive-to-active continuum. On the passive side is the individual who says if he were standing on the street corner and a bus jumped the curb and killed him, it would be okay. On the active side, the individual reports that the 3 o'clock bus comes by her street corner every afternoon. She has decided she will step off the curb in front of it tomorrow. Passive means individuals would just like to fall asleep and not wake up. Active means individuals are willing to use their energy to create a plan and implement it for their own demise (see Chapter 5).

Assessing a Reported Past Attempt:
If an attempt has occurred, it is important to assess the lethality (seriousness) of the attempt: **How** (was it attempted) + **Where** (was it attempted) = **Potential of Lethality**

The *How* of the attempt determines its potential reversibility. Refusing to eat for a day is different from ingesting a full bottle of pills; the type of pills taken is material to the potential lethality. The use of a firearm adds a further dimension of potential permanency to the suicide attempt.

The *Where* of the attempt impacts the potential for a rescuer to intervene. A woman who takes a handful of pills in front of her mother in the kitchen is much less likely to succeed in dying from the attempt than will a man who goes into the forest miles from anyone else, places a loaded handgun into his mouth, and pulls the trigger.

The suicidal chain of events then has several levels. These levels possess increasing detail and potential lethality:

Suicidal ideation

Suicidal ideation + Plan

Suicidal ideation + Plan + Intent

Suicidal ideation + Plan + Intent + Means

Suicidal ideation + Plan + Intent + Means + Attempt (assess the How and the Where)

The Big 1: The Chief Complaint

The final question moves to the individual's current problem, the chief complaint. Unless the individual is tearful, the clinician can accomplish several things by incorporating humor into the question, such as, "Other than the family car, what brought you in to see me today?" Asking the question in this way helps the clinician assess the individual's ego strength and ability to respond to a question that might evoke a smile; it continues to build rapport. If the individual is tearful, the question is straightforward: "What is bringing you in to see me today?"

As part of this section, the individual is asked to quantify his or her mood on a scale from 1 to 10, with 1 being the worst and 10 being the best. This gives a number that can be referred to in the future and reassessed at every session.

Documenting the Mental Status Exam:

Throughout the interview, the clinician needs to observe the individual for eye contact, facial expressions, movements, tics, recurrent coughs or sniffing (often a tic disorder), and/or recurrent behavior patterns.

The interview, including the MSE, is designed to paint a picture of the individual at a specific moment. Notes from this process will begin with a broad perspective of the individual, first painting the background onto the canvas. The chart documentation should:

❑ Describe the room in which the interview occurs. Is it in the clinician's office, the waiting room, or an emergency department setting?

❑ Describe the individual's mode of dress including shoes, socks, pants/skirt, shirt/blouse, and/or any other garments. Is the individual casually or stylishly attired? Are the colors coordinated? Is the individual wearing layers of clothing?

❑ Describe the individual's grooming. Is the individual neatly or merely adequately groomed? Is the individual disheveled? Is the individual lacking grooming skills?

- Describe the individual's demeanor. Is the individual cooperative, argumentative, or guarded?
- Describe the individual's speech patterns. Is speech smooth and flowing or hesitant? Is the speech staccato? How are the rate, rhythm, quantity, and amplitude of speech? Does the individual speak spontaneously or only respond to questions when asked? Are the answers short or complete sentences filled with information?
- Describe the individual's affect (see Box 1). Does the individual smile or cry? Is the affect bright or flat? Is the range of affect restricted or constricted, or does the individual demonstrate a full range? Is the individual's affect congruent with the stated mood?
- Describe the individual's thought processes:
  - Circumstantial – Does the individual begin logically and then meander around the answer and finally complete it?
  - Linear – Does the individual follow in a logical line?
  - Tangential – Does the individual begin to answer and then move into a completely different direction?
  - Thought blocking – Does the individual stop in midsentence and not continue with a given thought?
- Describe the individual's thought content. Are there any hallucinations, homicidal ideations, or suicidal ideations? Does the individual espouse any fixed, false beliefs (delusions)?

Included within the MSE are assessments of cognitive functioning, insight, judgment, and motor function/activity. This is not meant as an exhaustive approach to writing the MSE; it is meant to serve as a broad outline for assessing the individual's mental functioning.

Putting the MSE into Context

The initial purpose of the MSE is to assess the individual's:

- Appearance, behavior and speech
- Mood and affect
- Sensorium
- Intellectual function
- Thought content
- Thought processes
- Judgment
- Abstract ability
- Insight

Box 1. Affect Versus Mood

The terms *affect* and *mood* are often used interchangeably; technically, however, they are different. Affect is what the observer or interviewer objectively notes in an individual's demeanor. Mood is what the individual subjectively experiences and reports to the interviewer.

It is important for the clinician to assess whether the individual's stated mood is congruent with the affect that the clinician observes. If the 2 are not synchronous, this difference should be noted in the individual's record, eg, "Individual's stated mood is not congruent with observed affect." Individuals suffering from a thought disorder will often demonstrate an affect incongruent with the stated mood.

Ultimately, the examination allows the clinician to develop a diagnosis and formulate a treatment approach/plan for the individual.

Appearance, Behavior, and Speech. The clinician is observing and recording data with regard to the individual's attire and grooming. The clinician assesses how the individual relates to him or her, as well as looking for any eccentricities of speech in rate, rhythm, quantity, or amplitude. In appearance, the assessment looks at the type of clothing, clothing colors, the individual's grooming and hygiene, and indications of specific group affiliations based on clothing, colors, and tattoos. Certain styles of dress may connote personality disorders, such as histrionic personality disorder (see Chapter 6). Disheveled layering of clothing may lead to considerations of schizophrenia if other elements in the MSE are congruent with that diagnosis. Disturbances in speech may appear with rapid speech patterns and pressured speech, leading to suspicion of possible hypomania or mania. Does the individual demonstrate mutism as demonstrated by not speaking at all? Could it connote catatonic schizophrenia?

Mood and Affect. Mood is the individual's subjective description of how he or she is feeling, whereas affect relates to what the interviewer observes as the

The Goldman Guide to Psychiatry

individual's behavior. Ideally, affect and mood should be stable and consistent. Does the individual note that his or her mood remains constant or does it fluctuate from usual and customary (normal) to depressed? Does it go up and down or just have episodes into the elevated range? What is the range of the individual's affect? Is the affect flattened or blunted? Is the affect congruent with the individual's stated mood?

Sensorium. This section allows the clinician to assess for amnestic disorders, cognitive disorders, delirium, or dementia. It includes an assessment and description of the individual's orientation to person, place, time, and situation, as well as the individual's memory, ability to concentrate, and ability to perform mathematical calculations.

Intellectual Function. This section seeks to develop a sense of the individual's intellectual function and capacity. The questions probe the individual's use of vocabulary, skills in abstract thinking and mathematical functions, and ability to describe daily activities. In asking the individual to describe similarities between objects (How are a dog and cat similar?), the clinician obtains a sense of the individual's intellectual capacity and facility with abstract concepts. Some individuals will be very concrete in their thinking: The cat and the dog each have 4 legs. The individual with a greater intellectual capacity may be less concrete: The cat and the dog are pets. The individual who is more likely bright normal might respond: The cat and the dog are both mammals and can be domesticated (Box 2).

Of course, these questions give only a soft sense of the intellectual capacity of individuals. This may be adequate in many cases. If an actual diagnosis of intellectual functioning would be helpful in establishing a diagnosis and/or treatment approach, then a standardized intelligence test should be given. This type of testing is typically administered by psychologists trained in neuropsychological testing.

Thought. Two elements of thought, the process and the content, are assessed in the MSE. The clinician observes and determines if the individual's thought processes are coherent, logical, and goal directed (see Figure 1). Any of several categories of thought processes are likely to be observed:

- Circumstantial thought processes begin with the central theme and train of thought and meander through many detours, eventually returning to the central theme and reaching the desired goal in the conversation.

Box 2. Assessing Intellectual Function

The MSE provides a sense of the individual's intellectual function and capacity without benefit per se of actual intelligence testing. The individual's use of vocabulary, skills in abstract thinking and mathematical functions, and ability to describe daily activities, taken in combination reflect intellectual capacity. In particular, in asking the individual to describe similarities between common objects, the clinician obtains a "sense" of the individual's intellectual capacity for abstract thought. As noted above, a component of the MSE is asking the individual to describe similarities between:

- An apple and an orange
- A cat and a dog
- A knife and a fork
- A fly and a tree

Some individuals will be very concrete in their answers:

- The apple and the orange are round.
- The cat and the dog each have 4 legs.
- The knife and the fork have pointed ends.
- The fly and the tree, why, they aren't alike at all.

The individual with a greater intellectual capacity will be less concrete:

- The apple and the orange are fruit.
- The cat and the dog are pets.
- The knife and the fork are made out of metal.
- The fly and the tree, I don't know.

The individual who is more likely bright normal will respond:

- The apple and the orange have juice, taste sweet, and are healthy foods.
- The cat and the dog are both mammals and can be domesticated.
- The knife and the fork are eating utensils used to aid us in feeding ourselves.
- The fly and the tree are parts of nature and are living things.

While not producing hard numbers like those that result from intelligence tests, the MSE will provide a "soft," quick measure of an individual's intellect.

- Flight of ideas is demonstrated by thoughts rapidly jumping from one to another with a new central theme being introduced with each rapidly occurring thought. It is this jumping or racing of thoughts that may be indicative of attention-deficit/hyperactivity disorder, symptoms of hypomania and/or mania of bipolar disorder, schizoaffective disorder, or substance use.
- Linear thought processes move in a logical straight line, remaining true to the central theme and train of thought and directly answering the question asked.
- Loose associations of thought are sequentially disjointed or disconnected ideas. The listener is left confused as to the individual's meaning (may be indicative of bipolar disorder, delirium, dementia, substance use, or thought disorder).
- Tangential thought processes lose the central theme and train of thought and veer in different directions without ever returning to the original concept (may be indicative of bipolar disorder, dementia, substance use, or thought disorders).

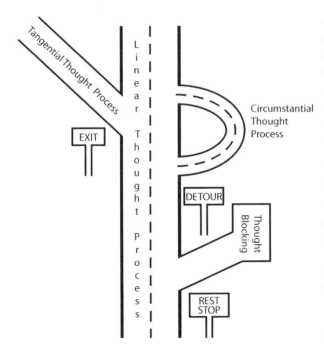

Moving in a straight line up and down the thought highway represents linear thought process. If one stops at a rest stop, meaning if one's thoughts seem to stop in mid stream as manifested by one's speech stopping in mid-sentence: thought blocking. If one seems to take a detour during the discussion, moving from the thought of the main highway to other thoughts, yet in the end comes back to the original theme: circumstantial thought process. If one seems to take an exit and go on to other ideas without ever coming back to the question or discussion at hand: tangential thought process. We make these determinations based upon the individual's use of speech and sentence content.

Figure 1. Goldman's Thought Highway.

- Thought blocking is observed when an individual abruptly stops speaking in mid-sentence. The individual does not finish the thought audibly, although he or she may complete the thought internally. On the other hand, the thought may remain incomplete (may be indicative of thought disorders).

Content. When the clinician performs the MSE, he or she assesses the individual's experience of hallucinations (perceptions without accompanying underlying auditory, visual, or tactile stimuli), and/or delusions (fixed, false beliefs). Misperceptions of actually occurring stimuli are illusions. Assessment of the individual's reported feelings of loneliness, rejection, or abandonment is another element in establishing his or her thought content.

Judgment. The individual's quality of judgment is assessed through the ability to make appropriate decisions. This assessment evaluates not only what individuals say they would do in a hypothetical situation; it evaluates as well what their history shows they have actually done. For example, if the clinician asked, "If you found an envelope on the ground that is stamped, sealed, and addressed, what would you do with it?" the expected response would be, "Well, of course, I would mail it." This response indicates the individual's judgment is intact. However, the individual's history may reveal multiple arrests for driving under the influence of either alcohol or an illicit substance, failing grades on the past 4 high school examinations, illicit substance use, or instances of driving the family car without a driver's license. Thus, it is important to look closely at individuals' general behaviors and recent activities to truly assess judgment. In other words, an individual saying he or she would mail the hypothetical envelope does not necessarily mean judgment is intact.

Abstract Ability. During the MSE, several questions evaluate the individual's abstractive ability, that is, the ability to think in deep and creative ways. In assessing an individual's abstractive skills and qualities, the clinician often obtains a clearer picture of the individual's intellectual capacity as well. When a clinician tests the individual's ability to describe similarities by asking the individual to compare apples and oranges, cats and dogs, knives and forks, and flies and trees, soft data is obtained as to the individual's intellectual capacity, which varies from concrete thinking to richer, more creative thought.

Insight. Insight allows human beings to understand their inner motivations, enabling them to look into themselves via "sight in." The process of therapy facilitates this inward sight, focusing on the individual's self-identity, feelings, and conflicts. Through the initial evaluation and the MSE, the clinician assesses the individual's understanding of his or her life situation, a gauge of the individual's baseline insight.

FINAL STEP IN THE INITIAL EVALUATION

After asking all of the questions and listening to the individual's chief complaint(s), the clinician concludes this first meeting with an important set of questions for the individual and/or family:

- What were you hoping I could do for you today?
- What were you hoping to achieve today?
- What is (or are) your expectation(s) of our working together?

The answers to these questions provide information crucial to subsequent actions in 2 ways. First, the psychiatrist/clinician can gauge the level of one element of individual insight: the individual's ability to recognize the current problem and to formulate a sense of what is needed to resolve it. Second, this information allows the clinician to understand what the individual hopes to achieve, whether the clinician can assist this individual, and whether this is an individual with whom the clinician feels therapeutically comfortable. In private practice, the psychiatrist may select those individuals with whom he or she wishes to proceed with treatment or decide to refer to someone else. If a relationship is established beyond the interview, the psychiatrist/clinician needs to determine if it will be as patient-clinician, as a consultant to the individual's primary care provider, or strictly as a second opinion.

The psychiatrist/clinician must assess the individual's expectations to know whether he or she will be able to meet them. Professionals must know their areas of expertise and their limitations. To paraphrase Socrates and Shakespeare, Know thyself and to thine own self be true. If the psychiatrist/clinician chooses not to establish a patient-clinician relationship, it is important to express this to the individual and to document the decision in the individual's chart.

CHAPTER THIRTEEN

Psychotherapy and Freud

THE FIVE AXES OF PSYCHIATRY

For each individual evaluated, the clinician makes 5 diagnoses, called the 5 axes. Each axis describes a separate quality or feature of the individual's illness(es). The 5 axes are as follows:

Axis I. Current Psychiatric Illness (State) – This defines the individual's current state of mind and deals with the acute condition of the individual psychiatrically (eg, major depressive disorder).

Axis II. Personality Disorder (Trait) – The personality is the matrix of all of the fibers of the fabric that makes up who the individual is. Thus, personality formation evolves over time; if there is in fact a disorder in the personality, it is a disruption in the smooth and orderly formation of the "who" the individual is. Personality disorders are not acute conditions; typically, they are chronic conditions that require long therapeutic introspection (insight) and treatment. Axis II is the place for recording personality disorder(s) and mental retardation (eg, histrionic personality disorder or borderline intellectual functioning).

Axis III. Medical Disorders (Physical Illnesses) – These are concurrent medical conditions with which the individual is dealing (eg, hypertension, fibromyalgia, diabetes mellitus, pneumonia).

Axis IV. Psychosocial Stressors (Social Disturbances) – These are the daily life issues impacting the individual, revolving around the trinity of: home, school/work, and/or recreation (eg, recent loss of employment, loss of a spouse, or a fire destroying the individual's home).

Axis V. Global Assessment of Functioning (Overall Ability to Function) – This is a numerical scale, found in the *Diagnostic and Statistical Manual for Mental Disorders, 4th Edition-TR*, that carefully categorizes the degree of disturbance in the individual's cognitive, psychiatric, and social life-functioning. The scale ranges from 0 to 100, with 100 equating to absence of distress and symptoms (eg, moderate symptoms with flat affect, circumstantial speech, and occasional panic attacks provide a score of 60).

After the initial interview and the Mental Status Examination are completed (see Chapter 12), the psychiatrist/clinician then formulates the following:

- A psychiatric differential diagnosis (typically, Axis I and Axis II)
- The 5 axes for this individual (complete diagnostic overview)
- A treatment plan
- Any plans for laboratory assessments
- Implementation of the treatment plan

Each of these is discussed fully with the individual and/or family members and informed consent obtained (see Appendix 1). Once agreement for treatment is reached, therapy can begin (Box 1).

Box 1. Transference and Countertransference

During therapy, the individual experiences an emotional and cognitive reaction to the therapist. This reaction is termed *transference*, because the individual is transferring feelings from past relationships onto the therapist and the treatment setting. The therapist also experiences emotional and cognitive reactions to each individual, referred to as *countertransference*. Assessing the individual's transference during therapy sessions enables the therapist to gain better therapeutic insight into the individual. On the other hand to provide the best and most professional care possible, the therapist must recognize and understand his or her own emotional and cognitive reactions to the individual (countertransference).

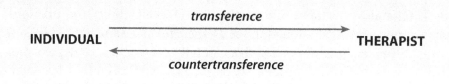

THERAPEUTIC OPTIONS

Current research and literature indicate that combination of psychotherapy and pharmacotherapy provides the richest results in treating psychiatric illness. Even in chronic thought disorders such as schizophrenia, the addition of psychotherapy in the form of cognitive behavioral therapy, family therapy, insight-oriented therapy, and individual supportive therapy can prove beneficial in helping the individual cope with the prospect and stressors of a life-long illness. Psychotherapy assists family members to develop appropriate skills to process and deal with the impact on the family of a life-altering illness. Multiple approaches are available in the arena of psychotherapy, which will only briefly be discussed in this chapter.

The issues that most often bring an individual to the psychiatrist fall into 3 broad categories:

- Issues having occurred in the remote past (often childhood)
- Issues pertaining to current psychosocial stressors
- Issues in the present that re-ignite past stressors, leading to current intrapsychic conflict

Some intrapsychic conflicts involve the individual alone, some involve the individual vis-à-vis others, and some relate to the family unit. A clinician takes a wide range of factors into account in assessing the individual to determine the appropriate treatment approach. The following list is an overview of psychotherapeutic approaches (see Appendix 5 for brief explanations):

- Behavior therapy
- Biofeedback
- Brief psychotherapy
- Cognitive therapy
- Crisis intervention
- Family therapy
- Group psychotherapy
- Hypnosis/hypnotherapy
- Marital therapy
- Psychoanalysis
- Psychodrama
- Psychodynamic psychoanalytic psychotherapy

These therapies may be used alone or in combination with other approaches, except for psychoanalysis (Box 2), which has a therapeutic exclusivity because of the intricate balance that is created in its application.

Box 2. The Birth of Psychoanalysis

Psychoanalysis was born out of treating the psychiatrically afflicted with hypnosis. Sigmund Freud and Josef Breuer were physicians treating individuals with hypnotic technique for neurologic disorders that did not conform to classical neurologic symptomatology. The case of *Anna O* [Bertha Pappenheim] is emblematic of the early hypnotherapeutic approach to treating intrapsychic conflict manifesting as somatic symptoms. Freud and Breuer noted that Anna O's symptoms of visual and motor dysfunctions disappeared during and after hypnotic trance, which the physicians postulated resulted from her verbalizations while in trance *(ventilating the intrapsychic conflict)*. The 2 physicians reported their findings in the now classic *Studies in Hysteria*, published in 1895.

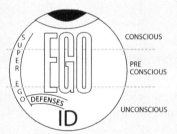

The hysteria of which they wrote has since come to be termed *conversion disorder*. They postulated that the condition resulted from a traumatic experience (usually of a sexual nature) that was too painful for the conscious mind; and the resultant unconscious conflict produced one or more physical manifestations. Freud believed the key to resolving the intrapsychic conflict was penetrating the unconscious resistance, which is managed by the unconscious defense mechanisms. Eventually, Freud forsook hypnosis for his newly developed technique of free association. Psychotherapy is based on Freud's structural concept of the mind components of id, ego, and superego and the concomitant topographic mind concepts of conscious, preconscious, and unconscious. Bringing these components together with the defense mechanisms provides an understanding of the process of intrapsychic conflict. Psychoanalysis became Freud's tool for treating the intrapsychic conflict and effecting resolution.

The Goldman Guide to Psychiatry

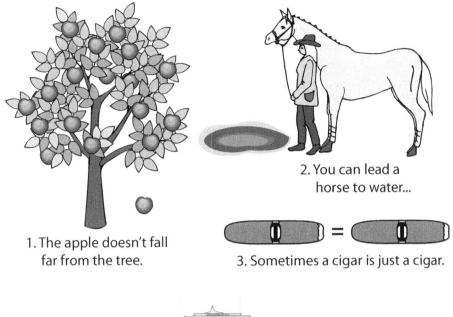

1. The apple doesn't fall far from the tree.

2. You can lead a horse to water...

3. Sometimes a cigar is just a cigar.

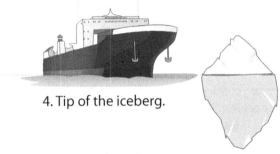

4. Tip of the iceberg.

Figure 1. Goldman's 4 Pictographs of Psychiatry

GOLDMAN ON FREUD

Goldman's 4 Pictographs of Psychiatry (Figure 1) present psychiatry in a nutshell. Pictograph 1 shows an apple tree with an apple falling to the ground, a depiction of the concept *The apple does not fall far from the tree*. We are all a product of both our nature and our nurture; we are guided by both our genetic make-up and the home in which we are raised. The genetic make-up is metaphorically the cards we are dealt, while our home of origin metaphorically determines how we will play that hand.

Pictograph 2 shows a woman holding the reigns of a horse near a stream, depicting *You can lead a horse to water; you cannot make him/her drink*. Our role as clinicians is to make an accurate diagnosis, formulate the appropriate treatment plan, and implement that plan. Unless the individual (and family) is committed to getting better, the level of success of the treatment plan may be sadly limited. If the individual chooses not to follow the medical recommendations when and where appropriate and accurate, the individual is unlikely to improve.

Pictograph 3 shows 2 cigars separated by an equal sign. Paraphrasing Freud, *Sometimes a cigar is just a cigar*. This admonishment serves to remind clinicians not to overanalyze individuals, situations, or themselves. Sometimes things happen out of sheer chaos or happenstance; there may not always be a dramatic psychoanalytic reason for a person's action.

Pictograph 4 shows an ocean liner and an iceberg, illustrating *The first time we meet an individual, all we see is the tip of the iceberg.* When the clinician meets an individual for the first time, the clinician observes only a small part of who that individual is. It is important to remember not to make a "snap" judgment—medical decisions must be based on an appropriate amount of accurate information. If we don't "look below the surface," we are at risk of running aground on the underlying shelf of the iceberg. We should avoid making a "shallow" assessment.

The Role of Insight in Psychotherapy

Psychotherapy is psychiatric surgery. It is no less painful than physical surgery and it is certainly no less invasive. It takes more time and many more sessions than surgical intervention because psychotherapy also encompasses the healing process in psychiatric disturbance.

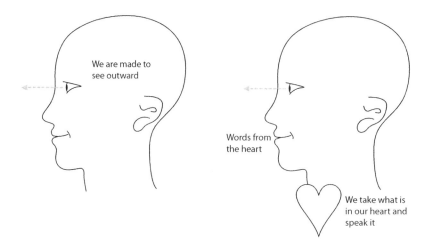

One of life's basic truths is that physiologically, human beings are built to "see out." They cannot see themselves without the benefit of a mirror. This is true of the inner psyche as well. If humans are made to see out, how do they see in? They must develop "sight in," that is, insight.

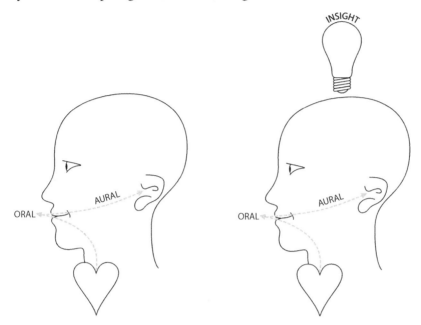

Humans gain insight by taking what is in their hearts (the emotional self) and verbalizing this by describing feelings; the verbalization moves from the mouth to the ears. By hearing what they are feeling, by saying what is "in their hearts", individuals are able to go from oral (spoken) to aural (heard). The information is heard, from mouth to ears, thus moving the verbalized information to the conscious mind, at which point they may experience the "Ah hah" phenomenon. The proverbial light bulb turns on. Through this process, individuals gain insight. Insight being sight into themselves, into their inner feelings and inner being. This allows the healing process to begin. (In the diagrams that follows, I utilize the eyeball as a metaphor for the individual seeking to "see" within him/herself. I place the Freudian components within the eye to highlight that while we are physiologically engineered to see out, through therapy we achieve the ability to see the self within).

Freud developed structural (id, ego, and superego) and topographical (conscious, preconscious, and unconscious) models that explain the mechanisms of the mind. These models underpin psychoanalytic efforts to help individuals gain insight. At birth, humans are essentially entirely id. Id is the primal energy that drives existence. Infants do 4 things well: eat, sleep, toilet, and cry. They do not distinguish between self and other. All exists for them alone. Then as they begin to mature, a new component of their being evolves, the ego.

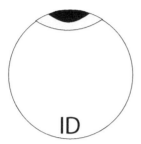 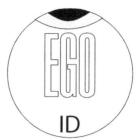

The ego is that component of their being that interacts with the outside world and brings about the new understanding that they exist as a separate entity. Through the ego, humans begin to understand the concepts of self and other, and the time frames of day and night, of past, present, and future. The evolving individual comes to comprehend that others do not exist solely for him or her.

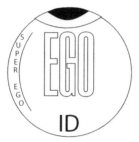 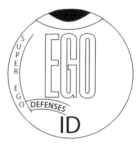

As individuals mature and evolve, another component evolves along with the id and the ego, the superego. The superego has been referred to as the internal policeman and policewoman, or as the internal 10 commandments: the internalized "thou shalts" and "thou shalt nots." The superego is the conscience, formed from parental guidelines and proscriptions; from society's rules, regulations, and perceived norms; and from religious precepts.

When the id, ego, and superego do not function in harmony, individuals experience internal strife called intrapsychic conflict. To resolve this unconscious intrapsychic conflict, a separate protective mechanism comes into play to keep this conflict from moving through the preconscious into the conscious mind: the defenses. The defense mechanisms serve to modify, neutralize, distort or negate the conflict in some way. Freud defined 7 defense mechanisms (see **Freud's Original 7 Defense Mechanisms** found on page 220).

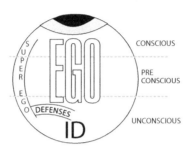

Freud's structural theory of the mind provides the mechanisms for the development of primal drives (id), self-identity (ego), the conscience (superego), and calming of intrapsychic conflict(s) (defense mechanisms). His topographical theory provides the levels/depths at which the machinations of the mind occur: activities of which we have full awareness (conscious); activities, feelings, thoughts, and concepts we access from memory (preconscious); and activities, feelings, thoughts, and concepts about which we are fully unaware (unconscious).

An Example of the Interplay of the Id, Ego, and Superego

It is 5:30 PM at the Jones house. The family will sit down to dinner promptly at 6:00 PM. Mom is home and Dad will arrive home shortly. Little Jimmy walks into the kitchen and finds one last chocolate mint cookie in the cookie jar. In his mind, the following internal exchange occurs:

> The Id: "Feed me."

> The Ego: "You know, I am hungry. It is that time of day when I usually eat. I think that cookie would be a great appetizer."

> The Superego: "Okay, guys. You both know better than this. Dinner is in about 30 minutes. Mom will really be upset, and Dad will back her up."

> The Id and the Ego: "Two out of 3, we are a democracy, so we prevail." Jimmy eats the cookie.

Mom walks into the kitchen, sees Jimmy by the empty cookie jar, and asks: "Jimmy! How could you eat just before dinner? How could you eat the last chocolate mint cookie when you know it is Dad's favorite?"

Jimmy looks up at Mom and says, "I didn't do it."

Mom takes Jimmy into the bathroom and stands him in front of the mirror where he can see the chocolate smudges and the crumbs all over his mouth and fingers.

Was Jimmy lying?

Intercession of the Defense Mechanism

The id, ego, and superego all exist within the unconscious realm of the mind. According to Freud, also residing in the unconscious are numerous defense mechanisms, which serve to modify, neutralize, distort or negate the facts in an effort to calm the intrapsychic conflict. As described in greater detail later, these mechanisms include:

- Denial – claiming or believing that what is true didn't happen
- Displacement – redirecting emotions to a substitute target
- Identification – defining self by identifying with others
- Projection – attributing uncomfortable feelings to others
- Reaction formation – overacting in the opposite way to the fear or conflict
- Repression – maintaining uncomfortable thoughts which are the product of intrapsychic conflict in the unconscious mind.
- Sublimation – redirecting socially inappropriate libidinal impulses into socially acceptable actions

In the example, Jimmy relies on the most common defense mechanism, denial. Intrapsychic conflict being unconscious, he is unaware of his behavior at the conscious level. If lying is a conscious act, then Jimmy was not lying when he told his mother he did not eat the cookie. The defense mechanism is activated because at his conscious level, the thought of losing Mom and Dad's love is so painful that the unconscious recruits the defense mechanism to negate this pain. Denying or negating the facts blocks the sensory data. Once Jimmy confronts the reality in the mirror of seeing the chocolate smudges and crumbs, the defense mechanism gives way to the conscious realities of guilt and shame, what might be called "psychiatric original sin." Individuals experience guilt for what they have done either by their actions or by the failure to act; shame arises from who they are or how they perceive themselves to be.

The personal computer offers a 21st-century metaphor for Freud's conscious, preconscious, and unconscious topographic layers of the mind (Figure 3). What is currently on the monitor's screen is the conscious mind, that is, what is presenting as the current reality. The preconscious mind is similar to the information on a diskette, zip disk, CD-ROM, or memory stick. To access that information, the individual types in a command via the keyboard; after several seconds, the information sought comes onto the monitor screen, to become the new reality. This is similar to what happens if someone asks, "Have you seen any good movies lately?" The response is, "Yes, I saw a great one last weekend. Give me a minute and I will be able to recall its name." After a moment, the name of the movie moves from the preconscious and enters the conscious mind and is spoken.

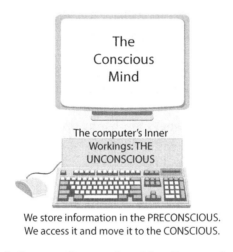

We store information in the PRECONSCIOUS.
We access it and move it to the CONSCIOUS.

Figure 3. Freud's 20th-Century Concept in a 21st-Century Analogy

Psychotherapy

Through therapy, individuals are able to develop an understanding of the interplay between the conscious, the preconscious, and the unconscious. With the assistance of a therapist who is trained to understand the language and meaning of intrapsychic conflicts, individuals come to make conscious sense of the unconscious conflicts. The therapist is the analog of the computer science specialist, who is trained in programming and repairing computer systems.

The Dream Trilogy

There are 3 types of dreams:

Patent dreams are dreams with clear meaning associated with a readily identifiable stimulus. Eg: during the day you step down from the sidewalk into the crosswalk and are almost struck by an oncoming car. That night you dream about the exact episode.

Latent dreams are dreams with garbled and confused meaning; they are the product of intrapsychic conflict. It is this type of dream that releases the intrapsychic energy.

Electrical discharge indicates dreams that are the result of the random firing of brain neurons during the sleep without meaning: similar to the flutter of an eyelid or the twitch of a finger.

Latent Dreams: The Royal Road to the Unconscious

Unlike the conscious and preconscious minds, the unconscious mind does not readily come onto the screen of awareness. When it does come into awareness via latent dreams, it does so in an unrecognizable code—the analog to computer programming languages such as COBOL and FORTRAN—so that it does not become readily understandable to the conscious mind. The unconscious is always functioning, even during sleep. Thus, in Freud's words, latent dreams are the "royal road to the unconscious." Latent dreams are disorganized screenplays that run in a person's mind during sleep. When a person is able to remember some of these dream sequences, they seem disjointed and unintelligible because they are coded in the language of the unconscious. Latent dreams serve as an outlet for energy generated at the unconscious level. The energy is the by-product of the intrapsychic conflict that needs to be released. Because elements of the inner conflict are too painful were they to be seen in the light of day of the conscious mind, the unconscious brings the elements to awareness in code via latent dreams.

The unconscious is analogous to a large steel drum, albeit a trash container. Everything we see, hear, feel, taste, smell, think, and experience goes into that container. Some of the experiences in our lives are fraught with moral and ethical dilemmas and lead to intrapsychic conflict. These conflicts seek to be resolved. They exert upward pressure, demanding to be heard.

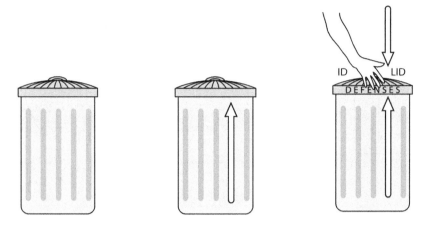

The lid of the trash container is symbolic of the defense mechanisms, or what I call "the id lid." The defenses seek to calm the intrapsychic conflict, maintaining it at the unconscious level, "protecting" the conscious from feeling the pain. In order to maintain the "id lid" in place requires a great amount of energy. This energy is very draining, and is often reported to the clinician as fatigue, excessive daytime tiredness, or generalized worry. Individuals will present with complaints of disturbance in sleep, appetite, memory, concentration, energy, and/or libido, all secondary to the diversion of energy to maintaining the id lid in place by engaging the use of the defense mechanism(s). Therapy is the process of placing a small tap into the bottom of the trash container and slowly releasing pieces of the intrapsychic conflict through the individual taking what is in his/her heart, converting these feelings into thoughts, these thoughts into words, and allowing those words into one's ears. Once heard, these thoughts convert from oral (spoken) to aural (heard), enter the brain, and allow insight to bring understanding of the conflict, achieving relief. As understanding evolves consciously (as insight is gained), the upward pressure from the unconscious intrapsychic conflict lessens, the pressure to maintain the id lid in place begins to release, and the individual experiences resolution in the conflict with improvement in the neurovegetative functioning inventory indices of sleep, appetite, memory, concentration, energy, and libido.

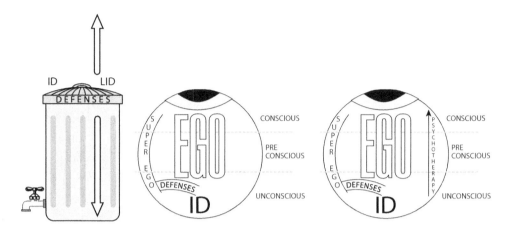

The tap (the therapeutic spigot), placed into the bottom of the container via therapy, is very gently opened at each therapy session, allowing the conflict to be slowly and steadily viewed by the individual in a very structured, safe, and guided manner. The spigot is the metaphor for talking therapy. The therapist is trained in knowing just how much to open the valve at each session; knowing just how evocative, supportive, and interventional to be. Remember that the conflict is occurring at the unconscious level. The process of psychotherapy allows the individual to gain conscious insight, allowing the unconscious conflict to leave the dark recesses of the unconscious mind, and come into the light of the conscious mind bringing healing and repair.

Freud's Original 7 Defense Mechanisms
As discussed above, Freud recognized that the interaction of the id, the ego, and the superego often creates an inner dissonance he called intrapsychic conflict. He identified the technique used by the mind at the unconscious level to calm this psychological upheaval as the defense mechanism. Freud detailed 7 defense mechanisms, which were later expanded by his daughter, Anna Freud, and categorized into a hierarchy by George Vaillant. Below is a thumbnail sketch of Sigmund Freud's original 7 defense mechanisms, all of which occur at an unconscious level.

Denial. The conflict between id, ego, and superego is resolved by the erasure of the awareness of the problem altogether. The conscious mind proceeds as if nothing ever happened. The external stimuli are actually blotted out from awareness (as in the example of Jimmy and the cookie).

Repression. This defense mechanism is a subtle variation of denial. In denial, the conscious awareness of the conflict is negated. In repression, the thought or conflict is either curbed before it reaches the conscious level (primary repression), or the idea, feeling, or conflict is excluded from awareness once it has reached the conscious level (secondary repression) (Box 3).

Box 3. Goldman's Theory of Somatic Consequences of Repression

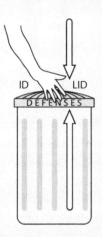

When the mind implements repression, a dramatic amount of energy is used to keep a lid on the unconscious. This effort is truly exhausting and requires real energy, the same energy needed to climb a long flight of stairs, to run several miles, or to work hard all day. This use of mind energy is energy-depleting and can cause a disruption in the sleep schedule, disturbance of appetite, disruption of memory and concentration, lack of energy (fatigue), and loss of libido. All of these complaints are heard when individuals describe the somatic side effects of depression and anxiety disorders. Somatization disorder and conversion disorder are key examples of this phenomenon. For so long as a lid is kept on the intrapsychic conflict, it does not become resolved. Repression prevents this conflict from rising into conscious awareness. Some of these conflicts, in pursuit of being "heard" will convert the body into their messenger and become a conversion disorder.

Projection. One way to understand projection is to think of the world as a collection of movie screens, and each person has a movie camera and projector. Individuals process everything happening around them and take that which is emotionally uncomfortable and shine it outside themselves onto other screens. To reduce inner conflict, an individual will take those uncomfortable and inappropriate inner impulses, feelings, and wishes and attribute them to someone else as being the other person's feelings, wishes, or impulses. For example, a man is late for an appointment and is driving too fast. Although the other drivers are traveling at the lawful speed limit, the rushed driver sees them as driving erratically. He becomes quite irritable. He begins to project onto the other drivers his emotional discomfort, commenting on how poorly they are driving. Hence, he takes his poor planning and erratic driving and projects them onto those around him. A second example might be of a young woman in a dating relationship who believes her partner is seeing someone else. She becomes jealous. When her boyfriend asks her how the relationship is doing, she tells him that he is asking this because he is jealous. She is attributing to her partner her own painful inner feelings, projecting her own insecurity onto her boyfriend.

Displacement. Figuratively speaking, when an individual is handed an emotional hot potato, he or she may attempt to hand it to someone else, thus using displacement to modify, neutralize, distort or negate the discomfort of intrapsychic conflict. Suppose when Henry goes to work tomorrow, his supervisor comes in sporting a foul mood. He calls Henry into his office and berates him for no apparent reason. Upset by this turn of events, on the way home that evening, Henry drives like a wild man, crowding other vehicles and frequently sounding his horn at the other drivers. When he walks in the front door of his home, his trusting dog, Rover, runs up to greet him, and Henry angrily pushes the dog out of the way. Have the other drivers done something to upset Henry or deserve his aggressive behavior? Has Rover done anything to deserve Henry's brusque and abrasive greeting? In fact, Henry is taking the negative energy given to him by his boss and displacing it onto the other drivers and Rover.

Identification. While identification can perform a positive, ego-building function by allowing children to incorporate word patterns or other mannerisms of their parents into their own repertoire of speech patterns and behaviors, as a defense mechanism it allows us to avoid dealing with painful emotions and intrapsychic dissonance. Separated from a loved one, for example, the individual identifies with an idealized view to calm feelings of loss, pain, or anxiety. An individual who is placed into the status of victim may take on the characteristics of the aggressor and in turn subjugate someone else. This mechanism improves the victim's sense of self-esteem by allowing him or her to rise above being the victim.

Reaction Formation. This defense mechanism takes an unconscious libidinal impulse and converts it to its direct opposite in conscious reality. For example, Henry has an incredible, insatiable libidinal impulse to spend time with prostitutes. Through the defense mechanism of reaction formation, he turns his impulse around by entering politics and ranting about the evil of prostitution. Henry seeks to get a city ordinance passed that will "clean up the streets once and for all."

Sublimation. This defense mechanism is a subtle variation of reaction formation. The individual still needs to defend against negative impulses. However, the impulse fulfillment is achieved via behavior that is socially acceptable, rather than socially objectionable. Once again, Henry has an incredible and insatiable libidinal impulse to spend time with prostitutes. Instead of ranting and railing against prostitution as in reaction formation, Henry turns the same libidinal impulse to its softer-edged, more positive expression via sublimation. He starts a social self-help organization for prostitutes to re-train and re-educate them to find new jobs that take them "off the street and out of harm's way."

CHAPTER FOURTEEN

Laboratory Tests and Scans in Psychiatry

The initial evaluation and the Mental Status Examination (Chapter 12) give information with regard to the individual's daily functioning and current life disturbances, leading to the development of a differential diagnosis. Before stating that the individual's disease is strictly supratentorial, that is, truly psychiatric, the clinician should rule out any underlying physiologic causes. This is achieved by obtaining a baseline of physiologic function with laboratory tests and values. When and where indicated, this laboratory assessment may include evaluation of adrenal function, electrolyte balance, glucose metabolism, kidney function, liver function, pancreatic function, and thyroid function. When indicated, it may be necessary to obtain a scan of the brain to rule out any space-occupying lesions or bleeding.

This chapter summarizes the basic approach to utilizing laboratory data in psychiatric care. This is a pragmatic clinical approach. Clinicians who suspect serious underlying physiologic, genetic, or toxic conditions should refer the individual to the appropriate specialist for evaluation and follow-up, including yet not limited to an allergy specialist, dermatologist, endocrinologist, gynecologist, infectious disease specialist, internist, neurologist, ophthalmologist, pulmonologist, radiologist, toxicologist, or urologist.

FIVE MAIN REASONS TO OBTAIN LABORATORY ASSESSMENTS

Laboratory tests may be needed before or during an individual's treatment for 5 main reasons:

1. To assess for an underlying physiologic or metabolic cause of the presenting psychiatric symptoms
2. To assess for the use of illicit substances as the cause of the presenting psychiatric symptoms

3. To establish a baseline of physiologic function before initiating a medication
4. To assess the safety and possible resultant side effect(s) of the medication(s) prescribed
5. To assess the therapeutic range of the medication prescribed

Lab Measurements to Assess Physical Causes of Psychiatric Disturbance

Disturbance in thyroid gland function may present with symptoms similar to either depression or hypomania/mania. Initial screening for thyroid-stimulating hormone (TSH) levels will help establish the presence of hypothyroidism (increased TSH) or hyperthyroidism (decreased TSH). If there is an abnormality in the TSH level, the individual should be referred to his or her primary care clinician or an endocrinologist for further evaluation.

A pheochromocytoma is a tumor of the adrenal gland, which may present with symptoms similar to anxiety or panic disorder. Measuring serum catecholamine or urine catecholamine levels can reveal this condition, at which point the individual should be referred to an endocrinologist.

Syphilis and human immunodeficiency virus (HIV) infection may present with cognitive disruption, confusion, depressed mood, hallucinations, and/or mood lability. Syphilitic paresis and acquired immunodeficiency syndrome dementia complex are the psychiatric components of these sexually transmitted disease states. If the individual might have a sexually transmitted disease, the clinician should obtain a Venereal Disease Research Laboratory (VDRL) test to screen for syphilis. If the VDRL result is positive, it should be confirmed with a specific fluorescent treponemal antibody-absorption test, which uses the spirochete *Treponema pallidum* as the antigen. Today, with appropriate permission obtained, clinicians are advised to order HIV testing for many of their individuals. The initial screening test for HIV is the enzyme-linked immunosorbent assay (ELISA), which if positive is then followed by the Western blot assay. While the ELISA is less expensive than the Western blot, it may give false-positive results. Thus, the sensitive and specific Western blot is utilized after a positive ELISA test result. It may be necessary to repeat the HIV test in individuals at high risk, such as intravenous drug users. An individual may have been exposed to the virus yet provide a negative HIV test result; he or she will not test positive until seroconversion has occurred. Seroconversion is the process whereby antibodies develop against an infectious agent and become detectable in the blood. With HIV, seroconversion usually occurs within 6 to 12 weeks after infection; however, in some cases it may take from 6 to 12 months for seroconversion to occur.

Seizure episodes may be preceded by auras that may be misinterpreted as hallucinations. The post-ictal state is one of confusion and mood changes that appears congruent with hallucinations, thought disorder, mood disorder/mood lability, and dementia. The primary assessment tool is an electroencephalogram (EEG). Measuring the serum prolactin level can assist in diagnosing the occurrence of a seizure if tested within 20 minutes of the putative seizure episode. In approximately 40% of seizure episodes, serum prolactin levels are elevated afterwards, providing a valid indication of a true seizure episode.

Liver dysfunction can result in hepatic encephalopathy manifesting with confusion and disturbance in thought processes. In individuals with these symptoms, the clinician should order assessment of serum ammonia levels to identify hyperammonemia, which is the culprit in hepatic encephalopathy. The following measures of liver function are useful:

- Alkaline phosphatase and gamma-glutamyltranspeptidase (GGT) to assess for an obstruction in the biliary system either within the liver itself or outside the liver in the bile channels
- Alanine aminotransferase (ALT) and aspartate aminotransferace (AST) to assess liver cell damage
- Lactate dehydrogenase (LDH) and total bilirubin (bilirubin is a breakdown product of hemoglobin)

Infectious diseases with fever can result in changes in consciousness and cognitive function congruent with mood, thought, or cognitive disorders. A baseline complete blood cell count (CBC) can indicate an infection when the white blood cell count is elevated.

It is often prudent to obtain a urine pregnancy test in women of childbearing age. Pregnancy impacts mood and thought processes. It is also important to assess for pregnancy when obtaining an x-ray, CT scan, or initiating medication for this population.

It is valuable to assess vitamin and mineral levels. Nutritional deficiencies can masquerade as psychiatric disorders. Deficiencies in Vitamin B complex (most notably B1, B6 and B12) and folate can present with fatigue, disruption in memory and concentration, and disturbance in mood. Vitamin D deficiency can present with symptoms similar to fibromyalgia. Obtaining lab values of Vitamins A and D is also important due to the potential to receive too much of these fat soluble vitamins.

For men and women 45 years old or older, it is beneficial to obtain sex hormone levels. Men who present with fatigue, loss of libido, and/or loss of motivation, who suspect depression, might be suffering from low testosterone levels. Women may be perimenopausal.

Ruling Out Illicit Substance Use

Obtaining a urine drug screen is appropriate before initiating therapy to establish a diagnosis of substance abuse disorder. In addition, this test is indicated anytime during therapy if behavior or cognitive changes occur. Telltale signs of illicit substance use/abuse may be detected in the urine within specified time frames (Table 1).

Table 1. Time Frame Within Which Illicit Substances Are Detectable in Urine

Substance	Detectable Time
Alcohol	7–12 hours
Amphetamine	48 hours
Benzodiazepine	72 hours (3 days)
Benzodiazepine metabolites	48–96 hours (2–4 days)
Cannabis sativa (marijuana)	72 hours to 30 days
Cocaine	6–8 hours
Codeine	48 hours
Heroin	36–72 hours
Methadone	72 hours
Phencyclidine (PCP)	112 hours (8 days)

Obtaining a Baseline Assessment

Before the clinician starts an individual on a medication, he or she is wise to obtain baseline serum (blood) levels first. This fulfills 3 main functions:

1. It allows the clinician to rule out possible physical illnesses that may underlie the psychiatric issues and/or illnesses that may be comorbid with the psychiatric disturbance.
2. Should the clinician need to switch to another medication later, initial baseline laboratory values are already available, eliminating a delay in prescribing the new medication.
3. The clinician can assess the individual's physiologic response to the medication based on the pre-medication baseline laboratory values.

Generally, baseline testing will include:

- CBC with platelet count and reticulocyte count
- TSH
- Liver function tests, i.e., AST, ALT, LDH, alkaline phosphatase, total bilirubin
- Amylase, lipase (baseline pancreatic function)
- Blood urea nitrogen/creatinine (BUN/Cr) (kidney function)
- Serum electrolytes checking for baseline potassium, sodium, calcium, chloride, bicarbonate, and glucose (monitoring for possible diabetes mellitus)
- Electrocardiogram (ECG)
- Urine pregnancy test in female individuals aged 11 to 45 years who have begun menstruation and have not had a hysterectomy or passed through menopause

Assessing Safety and Side Effect Profile

Antipsychotic Medications. Antipsychotic medications can cause leukocytosis, leukopenia, and/or agranulocytosis. Thus, the CBC test is very important, first as a baseline and then during pharmacotherapy, to assess for any hematologic adverse effects. Individuals on antipsychotic medications can develop neuroleptic malignant syndrome, the symptoms of which include confusion, muscle stiffness, hypertension/hypotension, and/or hyperpyrexia. If neuroleptic malignant syndrome is suspected, levels of creatinine phosphokinase (CPK) should be measured. Typically, the creatinine phosphokinase level will begin to elevate as the syndrome begins, continuing to rise until grossly elevated (normal is 5–50 IU/L). A weekly white blood cell count is required when Clozaril (clozapine) is prescribed, because of the potential for agranulocytosis (1%–2% incidence). Agranulocytosis is characterized by a dramatic decrease in the number of circulating neutrophils, leading to the inability to successfully defend against infections. It is important to monitor individuals taking atypical antipsychotics for the symptoms of metabolic syndrome. The indicia to monitor are blood pressure, fasting plasma glucose, high-density lipoprotein cholesterol, triglycerides, and waist circumference. In order to appreciate the gravity of the lab value results, it is valuable to have baseline labs and blood pressure values that were obtained prior to initiating the atypical antipsychotic medication.

Tricyclic Antidepressants. Tricyclic antidepressants (TCAs) have the potential to slow the conduction of electrical impulses through the cardiac muscle, so ordering a baseline ECG is good practice to rule out any preexisting cardiovascular disease and to provide a baseline for an individual who is later prescribed a TCA. A follow-up ECG can be compared with the baseline ECG to provide evidence of any cardiac adverse effects from the TCA.

When prescribing imipramine in children for attention-deficit hyperactivity disorder, anxiety, depression, or enuresis, it is prudent to obtain a serum level of the medication. Measuring serum levels of Norpramin (desipramine) and Pamelor (nortriptyline) assists in maintaining dosing within the therapeutic window and preventing toxic dosages (Table 2).

Table 2. Therapeutic Ranges for Tricyclic Antidepressants and Major Mood Stabilizers

Medication	Therapeutic Level
Depakote (divalproex/valproate)	50–100 µg/mL
Elavil (amitriptyline)	100–250 µg/mL
Lithobid, Eskalith (lithium)	0.5–1.5 mEq/L
Norpramin (desipramine)	150–300 µg/mL
Pamelor (nortriptyline)	50–150 µg/mL
Sinequan (doxepin)	100–250 µg/mL
Tegretol (carbamazepine)	4–12 µg/mL
Tofranil (imipramine)	150–300 µg/mL

Major Mood Stabilizers. When the clinician first prescribes a major mood stabilizer for an individual, it is prudent to obtain baseline laboratory values.

- **Depakote (divalproex sodium/valproic acid).** Divalproex sodium can adversely impact the reticulocyte count, the liver, and the pancreas, and has a therapeutic serum range. It is good practice to obtain baseline CBC with a reticulocyte count and platelet count before initiating this medication, along with a baseline liver profile and amylase and lipase levels. Serum levels should be assessed during upward titration of the medication; the CBC with reticulocyte and platelet counts, and pancreas and serum levels should be repeated every 3 months for the first 2 years, then every 6 months thereafter.

- **Lithium**. This medication clears through the kidneys and can adversely affect kidney function. It can also elevate the white blood cell count and affect electrical tracings on an ECG. Lithium can adversely impact thyroid functioning, leading to hypothyroidism. In a pregnant woman, lithium can adversely impact the gestating fetus, causing the cardiac condition Ebstein's anomaly in the first trimester. Thus, the clinician should order a serum beta human chorionic gonadotropin test or a urine pregnancy test in women of childbearing age before initiating lithium therapy. The serum level of lithium has a narrow therapeutic range of 0.5mEq/L to 1.2mEq/L. The recommended laboratory tests for lithium are a BUN/Cr, CBC, serum lithium level, and TSH every 3 months for the first year, then every 6 to 12 months each year thereafter.

- **Tegretol (carbamazepine)**. This medication is similar to divalproex sodium/valproic acid in its potential risks and side effects. It is good practice to obtain a baseline CBC with a reticulocyte count and platelet count before initiating therapy, along with a baseline liver profile and amylase and lipase tests. It is important to assess serum carbamazepine levels during upward titration of the medication and to repeat laboratory tests for liver function, CBC, pancreas function, and serum levels every 3 months for the first 2 years, then every 6 months thereafter. The therapeutic range is 4 µg/mL to 12 µg/mL.

- **Trileptal (oxcarbazepine)**. A medication that is often used off-label for mood stabilization, oxcarbazepine can affect sodium levels, so it is important to check periodically for a decrease in sodium (hyponatremia).

- **Topamax (topiramate)**. Topiramate is used on label prophylactically for migraine headaches or off-label to produce weight loss and to stabilize mood. If individuals complain of eye pain, tonometry to check intraocular pressure is indicated, as a possible adverse effect of this medication is acute myopia and angle closure glaucoma.

IMPORTANT LABORATORY KEY POINTS

- When ordering laboratory tests, the clinician should ask to have the performing laboratory include the reference ranges with all results. These ranges indicate the limits of what is normal, meaning what is acceptable or what is referred to as *within normal limits*.

- If an individual's results come back *out of range*, either high or low, confirm that the laboratory is using the proper reference range. If the individual is a child, for example, the reference range provided may be keyed for adults. In such a case, the clinician should consult a pediatric text for appropriate pediatric/non-adult laboratory reference ranges. This prevents any misunderstanding for the individual and/or his or her parents with regard to the laboratory results. Before a clinician reports ECG results to an individual or the individual's parents or guardian, the clinician should confirm that the report is a confirmed report. A confirmed report is one that has been reviewed by the laboratory's cardiologist, who has approved the results.

- If the results seem to be inconsistent with past laboratory results, the clinician should order a repeat of the tests. Laboratory errors can and do occur. Hemolysis, the breakdown of red blood cells, can occur when samples have been improperly stored prior to or during transport. The specimen may not have contained enough volume to provide the necessary amount for an accurate test result.

- While it is acceptable to call the laboratory for initial results, the clinician should obtain a printed copy of the results to place into the individual's medical record.

After obtaining the laboratory results, the clinician should review the results with the individual or the individual's parents or guardian at the next appointment, documenting in the medical record that the results were reviewed. If the results are outside of the reference range and indicate the need for further medical workup or change in medication, the individual or the individual's parents or guardian should be contacted as soon as possible and the conversation noted in the individual's medical record.

DIAGNOSTIC SCAN PROCEDURES

Computerized Tomography (CT)

Unlike the traditional x-ray machine that sends a single beam through the body, the CT device sends several beams through the body simultaneously from different angles. These beams are then detected and their strength is measured. Beams passing through less dense tissue such as vital organs show up stronger than beams that pass through denser tissue such as bone. A computer processes these results and displays the results as a 2-dimensional display on a monitor screen. The CT scan allows for assessment of brain tissue to rule out intracranial bleeding and space-occupying lesions, as well as aneurysms and abscesses. Individuals who present with sudden-onset disturbances in behavior and/or cognitive function should undergo CT scanning of the head to rule out cerebral vascular accidents and/or space-occupying lesions.

Magnetic Resonance Imaging (MRI)

The MRI device uses radiofrequency waves and a magnetic field to produce its images. The MRI scan provides clear pictures of soft-tissue structures without radiation. MRI scans of the head are useful in ruling out space-occupying lesions, changes in the ventricles, and/or multiple sclerosis.

Positron Emission Tomography (PET)

The PET scan relies on the detection of radiation that is emitted from a radio-active substance ingested by or injected into the individual. The radioactive substance, which emits small particles called positrons, localizes in the desired area of assessment and is detected by the PET scanner. The substance is visual-ized as different colors and/or degrees of brightness, which allows the reading clinician to understand the level of tissue or organ function. PET scanning is effective is assessing function in specific areas of the brain.

Single Photon Emission Computed Tomography (SPECT)

SPECT scanning combines CT scanning with a radioactive tracer, which allows the physician to observe blood flow through the tissues and organs. Unlike the PET scan, the radioactive-labeled tracer in SPECT scanning stays in the bloodstream, rather than being absorbed by nearby tissues. This allows SPECT scans to provide views of areas of blood flow. SPECT scans are best used in assessing blood flow through arteries and veins in the brain.

X-ray Examinations

X-ray examinations assess for irregularities in the bony components of the body and are used to identify injury to the bones of the skull.

APPENDIX 1

Informed Consent

Informed consent must be obtained before initiating any medication or treatment approach. Informed consent means exactly what the 2 words imply. The individual must be informed of risks, side effects, and benefits in terms that he or she clearly understands. The individual must also be advised of the possible outcome(s) if he or she chooses not to undergo the procedure or utilize the medication. Then the individual can either give consent for treatment or make the informed decision to refuse treatment. For complete informed consent, the individual must also be informed of the possibility of alternative treatments. The informed consent scenario should be included in the individual's medical record.

What follows is an example of what might be charted when informed consent or informed refusal is obtained:

INFORMED CONSENT

"I discussed with the patient/parent/guardian the risks and side effects of the medication/procedure, [name of medication(s)/description of the procedure(s)], as well as potential benefits, and discussed the following risks and side effects, including yet not limited to: [before prescribing an antipsychotic medication, for example, the clinician would discuss akathisia, dystonic reaction, metabolic syndrome, neuroleptic malignant syndrome, parkinsonian-like tremor, and tardive dyskinesia]. I also explained the potential outcome(s) if the procedure is not undertaken/the medication is not taken. The patient/parent/guardian expressed understanding in his or her own words of the information given, and expressed this understanding in terms congruent with all that I had discussed. The patient/parent/guardian gave informed consent for initiation of [name of medication(s)/name the procedure] at [initial dose of medication] with upward titration as clinically indicated."

INFORMED REFUSAL

"I discussed with patient/parent/guardian the potential risks of not initiating treatment; the patient/parent/guardian expressed understanding congruent with my explanation and stated his or her desire to:

❑ defer treatment
   or
❑ refuse treatment

at this time."

When possible, the clinician should demonstrate the possible side effects that lend themselves to a visual presentation. For clinicians who choose to give individuals printed handouts for each of the medications prescribed or procedure(s) recommended, the handouts do not take the place of discussing the risks and side effects of the medication(s) and procedure(s) face-to-face with the individual. If printed handouts are provided, document in the chart that the individual received them. This shows that the individual received a second form of information to support the informed consent or the informed refusal.

Explanations must be in plain, clear language. If the individual is not fluent in English, someone conversant in the individual's native language must be available to translate clearly for the individual what has been explained. The individual should repeat to the interpreter what was said to verify his or her clear understanding. This applies also to individuals who are deaf.

Individuals should be told that if a serious side effect occurs, they must go immediately to the nearest emergency department and have their clinician paged from there. With the individual in a safe setting, the clinician can maintain continuity of care and address immediate care needs by speaking with the emergency staff.

When individuals refuse a medication or procedure, the clinician should explain the prognosis for the condition when not treated. Alternative therapeutic approaches, if any, should be mentioned. When applicable, the clinician should direct the individual to the appropriate practitioner to provide alternative services, if available and if requested by the individual. When available and when requested, offer the individual several names of competent practitioners from which to choose.

APPENDIX 2

Inducing Sleep

When individuals present to the clinician with the complaint of not being able to sleep, the clinician should ask the following questions about sleep:

- What time do you typically go to bed at night?
- What time do you typically fall asleep?
- Do you have difficulty initiating sleep?
- Do you have difficulty maintaining sleep?
  - If you have arousals during the night's sleep, how many do you have?
  - If you arouse from sleep, are you able to go back to sleep?
  - If you are able to go back to sleep, how long does it take from arousal to falling back to sleep?
- Do you have difficulty awakening in the morning at the appropriate time?
- Do you awaken at the same time every morning?
- How many hours of sleep do you typically receive each night?
- When you awaken, do you feel rested or do you still feel tired?
- When did your sleep disturbance begin?

For individuals having difficulty initiating sleep at night, the clinician should evaluate for narcolepsy, obstructive sleep apnea/hypopnea syndrome, and shift work sleep disorder. Also review the individual's current medication regimen to determine if any of his or her medications are adversely impacting sleep. Assess for mood disorders, anxiety disorders, and thought disorders as culprits for sleep disruption. If these are ruled out, the diagnosis is most likely primary insomnia. The first step is to assess the individual's sleep habits and to review sleep hygiene. The major components of effective sleep hygiene are:

- Going to bed at the same time every night
- Arising at the same time every morning
- Using the bed for sleep and intimacy only
- Maintaining the ambient temperature in the bedroom at a comfortable level for the individual
- Maintaining the light levels in the bedroom at a comfortable level for the individual

- Maintaining sound levels in the environment at a level that is sleep enhancing, not sleep disrupting
- Not eating for several hours before initiating sleep
- Not drinking liquids for several hours before initiating sleep
- Discontinuing the use of alcohol until a regular sleep pattern is established (use is then reassessed)
- Discontinuing the use of caffeine until a regular sleep pattern is established (use is then reassessed)

After sleep hygiene has proven ineffective in restoring sleep or establishing comfortable sleep initiation and a renewable pattern of sleep, the algorithm for prescribing sleep-inducing medication is as follows:

1. Rozerem (ramelteon)
2. Sonata (zaleplon)
3. Lunesta (eszopiclone)
4. Ambien/Ambien CR (zolpidem tartrate/extended release)

Rozerem (ramelteon) was approved by the US Food and Drug Administration (FDA) in 2005 to induce sleep in individuals with insomnia. Unlike other sleep-inducing medications, ramelteon does not bind to the gamma-amino butyric acid ($GABA_A$) receptors. It is a melatonin receptor agonist that targets the melatonin$_1$ and melatonin$_2$ receptors found in the suprachiasmatic nucleus of the hypothalamus. This nucleus serves as the master clock for the circadian rhythm cycles. Ramelteon is the only non-scheduled prescription medication FDA approved for sleep induction. It is noted not to have abuse potential, rebounding insomnia potential, or withdrawal symptoms. It is dosed as 8 to 16 mg by mouth 30 minutes to 1 hour before bedtime. It is taken for 10 to 12 nights before its effectiveness is assessed. Because of its mechanism of action and approval for long-term use without abuse, rebounding insomnia, or withdrawal symptoms, this medication serves as a good first-line treatment approach. If it does not prove effective, then the next approach is the clinically short-acting Sonata (zaleplon).

Sonata (zaleplon) was FDA approved in 1999. While not a benzodiazepine, its site of action is at the type$_1$ benzodiazepine receptor on the $GABA_A$ complex within the central nervous system. The onset of action is approximately 30 minutes after ingesting the medication, and duration of action is approximately 4 hours. Zaleplon has a half-life of 1 hour, which means it may be used to initiate sleep and to re-initiate sleep should the individual awaken during the night. The medication clears the system quickly so the individual typically does not suffer a "hang over" effect on awakening.

Lunesta (eszopiclone), FDA approved in 2004 for the treatment of insomnia, is a hypnotic with a chemical structure different from the benzodiazepines. It is an agonist at the benzodiazepine receptor, binding selectively at the $omega_1$ receptor site. Eszopiclone induces sleep without the anxiolytic qualities of the benzodiazepines. It has a half-life of 6 hours. Eszopiclone is the only category IV controlled substance FDA approved sleep-facilitating medication currently approved for long-term use of 3 to 6 months.

Ambien (zolpidem tartrate) is a hypnotic/sedative approved by the FDA in 1993 for inducing sleep in individuals experiencing insomnia. The medication binds with high affinity to the $alpha_1$ $GABA_A$ subunit receptors. It is approved for short-term use (2 weeks to 6 weeks). While it has a half-life of 2 to 3 hours, there have been reports of morning hang-over, nighttime sleepwalking, sleep eating, sleep spending, and unremembered sexual activity. For most individuals, it is a safe and effective treatment for insomnia. Zolpidem is used by the US Air Force to help pilots sleep in their downtime [and the stimulant Provigil (modafinil) is prescribed when military pilots need to be focused, alert, and awake]. In 2005 the FDA approved the longer acting form of Ambien CR. It is a bilayer medication with a short-acting, immediate-release layer followed by the longer-acting layer.

When the algorithm of Rozerem, Sonata, Lunesta, Ambien does not prove effective, the next approach is to utilize medications with greater potential for side effect while the medications have a great potential for effecting the induction of sleep:

Chloral hydrate was first discovered in 1832, and has been inducing sleep since 1869. It is available as a brand as either Somnote or Noctec. Chloral hydrate is given as either an oral solution or as a capsule. It is given from 500mg to 2000mg. It is for short term use. Long term use can result in tolerance, dependence, and/or withdrawal – the components of abuse. When given for too long a period of time, liver damage can occur. An overdose can prove fatal.

Clonidine, an $alpha_2$ agonist, is used off-label to facilitate sleep in children and adolescents. For children and adolescents utilizing clonidine adjunctively with a psychostimulant in treating ADHD, the child/adolescent often will receive a dose of the clonidine at bedtime to facilitate sleep. Some individuals will experience a decrease in mood secondary to clonidine. Some will experience nightmares from clonidine as a paradoxical response, as it is often given off-label to calm nightmares and induce sleep. Clonidine is given to offset aggressive acting out in ADHD and is dosed from 0.1mg per day up to 0.4mg per day, in divided doses.

Remeron (mirtazapine) is an antidepressant medication that provides sedation at its lower dosing range. Remeron is available as 15mg, 30mg, and 45mg. The 15mg caplet may be broken in half into two 7.5mg parts. The 7.5mg proves most sedating. It is the antihistaminergic moiety that is more pronounced at the 7.5mg dose and the 15mg dose. It is this antihistaminergic component that provides the sedation, as well as appetite/weight gain enhancement. This is an off-label use of this medication.

Seroquel (quetiapine) is an atypical antipsychotic medication that is gaining favor among psychiatrists in treating anxiety and insomnia – using the medication off-label and in low doses. The quetiapine is dosed at 25 to 50mg to induce sleep. While its dosing range allows for up to 800mg per day for Schizophrenia, for sleep it is typically not dosed beyond 100mg at night.

Trazodone, an heterocyclic antidepressant, has been used off-label for inducing sleep since the 1980's. It was used in combination with Prozac (fluoxetine) when fluoxetine was first introduced in 1988. The fluoxetine was given in the morning for depressive disorder, and the Trazodone was given at night to offset any insomnia side effects from the fluoxetine. It is typically dosed at 25mg to 50mg at bedtime. Its most notable serious potential side effect is priapism: a painful, prolonged erection that may be a medical emergency.

APPENDIX 3

Two Words to Avoid in Therapy:
BUT and WHY

In therapy, as well as in life, I avoid two words: But and Why. The reason for avoiding these words is very powerful.

The word **BUT** negates all that comes before it. Parents regularly communicate conditional love by saying to their children: "I love you, but when you do x (whatever that behavior is), I get very angry." The end result is that the parent has said: "I love you <u>until</u> you engage in that behavior" or "I love you <u>except</u> when you engage in that behavior." The parent has essentially told the child that the child is not loved when that behavior occurs. The parent has created conditional love.

The correct way to approach unwanted behaviors: "I love you. [period] When you engage in this behavior, I am unhappy with the behavior. Let's talk about this." Note, the period after "I love you." That communicates the parent's love to the child, period. Then the parent expresses dissatisfaction with a specific behavior, NOT with the child.

This relates to any and all use of the word BUT. "I enjoyed the movie, but I didn't like the part about…." communicates that the person didn't really enjoy the movie. And on it goes.

The word **WHY** is overwhelming to individuals. It is asking 5 questions at one time: How, What, When, Where, and Who? That overwhelms the individual, causing the person to engage his/her unconscious defense mechanisms immediately. When someone is asked, "Why did you do that?" The person feels immediately on the defensive. Instead of asking "Why?", take the time to ask the individual each component of the situation:

- How did this come to pass?
- What do you think led to this result?
- When did this occur?

- Where did this come from? or Where did this take place?
- Who was involved with you? or Who was affected by this?

In so doing, you allow the individual to sort through the process and to gain valuable insight into how the situation occurred, what each step of the occurrence was, when it occurred, where all of the components came from, and with whom and to whom connectivity exists with regard to the incident.

You will notice in my text, THE GOLDMAN GUIDE TO PSYCHIATRY, neither of these two words is used, except in the Folstein Mini Mental State Exam when the individual is asked to repeat the phrase: "No ifs, ands, or buts."

APPENDIX 4

Augmenting Antidepressant Therapy

There are occasions when antidepressant medication(s) need assistance or modification:

1. The medication does not provide full effectiveness
2. The medication is effective and causes side effect(s)
3. The medication is effective and then loses its effectiveness
4. The medication treats one of a constellation of illnesses (comorbidities) and not all of the symptoms being experienced

1. <u>The medication does not provide full effectiveness</u>. When individuals report partial benefit from an antidepressant, the question arises as to how much benefit is derived: 10%, 20%, 50%, 75%? Typically partial benefit is due to improper dosing of the medication. Often upward titration of the medication will enhance the benefit received. Once the medication has been titrated to its upper limit and benefit is still not complete, the next step is to reassess the diagnosis. For so long as the diagnosis is accurate, the next step is to reassess the medication. If the medication is properly indicated, before changing it to another medication either within its family or to another family of medications, one must reassess for adjunctive therapy: the addition of another medication to enhance the benefit of the first. Below are listed the adjunctive/augmenting approaches:

- Atypical Antipsychotic medications
- Deplin (L-Methylfolate)
- Lithium
- Nontraditional psychostimulant (modafinil)
- Traditional psychostimulants (amphetamine, methamphetamine, methylphenidate)
- Thyroid stimulating therapies (synthroid, cytomel)
- Wellbutrin XL (bupropion) added to an SSRI to augment the serotonin benefit with dopamine and a small amount of norepinephrine

Atypical antipsychotic medications are currently being added to antidepressant treatment when the antidepressant alone does not bring full relief from the depressive disorder. While the mechanism of action is not fully understood, it is possible that the depressive disorder is actually a subset of a bipolar illness. In such an instance, the antidepressant medication improves the mood while the atypical antipsychotic medication stabilizes the mood. While all of the atypical antipsychotic medications are FDA approved for treating bipolar disorder, Abilify (aripiprazole) was approved in November 2007 for adjunctive antidepressant use, and in March 2009 Zyprexa (olanzapine) was approved in combination with Prozac (fluoxetine) [the combination medication Symbyax] for treating treatment resistant depression (TRD) and for the acute treatment of bipolar depression.

Deplin (L-methylfolate) is the component of folate that is able to cross the blood brain barrier and serves as the catalyst substrate for rebuilding and replenishing the supply of bioamine neurotransmitters in the presynaptic neurons. The antidepressants block the presynaptic reuptake transport pump, or block the disassembly of the returned neurotransmitter, or release the brake from the presynaptic autoreceptor thus freeing the release of neurotransmitter into the synapse, or perform a combination of any two or all three. When an antidepressant medication is only partially effective, it is possible that it is fully performing its function, while the presynaptic neuron is unable to build new neurotransmitter. Thus the reuptake pump has nothing to block, monoamine oxidase has nothing to disassemble, and releasing the autoreceptor brake releases nothing into the synapse. Adding in Deplin replenishes the neurotransmitter supply so that the antidepressant medication's mechanism of action can provide its intended benefit. Deplin is an FDA approved medical food. It is provided by prescription only. It is as safe as a vitamin and as potent as a medication. It is dosed as 7.5 mg once per day. It may be increased to 15 mg per day if necessary.

Lithium is an alkali metal found on the periodic table as a naturally occurring element. In its salt form it is used to stabilize mood. It first came into medical use in 1948 under the auspices of John Cade, MD, for treating bipolar disorder. Lithium was banned in the United States until 1970 when it was approved for use. While it typically must stay within a specified serum level to provide benefit for bipolar disorder (0.5mEq/L to 1.2mEq/L), it is used at smaller doses for augmenting antidepressant medication(s) for treating partial responses. Its mechanism of action is not well understood. It may be that the true diagnosis is a subtype of bipolar disorder and the lithium assists in treating the bipolar component. It may be that the lithium calms the underlying anxiety, thus allowing an improvement in mood. For some individuals, this is a beneficial augmentation.

Non-traditional Stimulant Provigil (modafinil) is an energy-enhancing medication that is currently FDA approved for excessive daytime sleepiness associated with narcolepsy, obstructive sleep apnea/hypopnea syndrome, and shift-work sleep disorder. It is currently used off-label to offset the residual sleepiness and fatigue that often occur in depressed individuals. It is used adjunctively off-label to enhance the mood benefits of antidepressant medications. It has benefit for reestablishing energy and improving focus and concentration. For individuals with a milder variant of depression not meeting the criteria for major depressive disorder, modafinil is being used off-label to treat what is being called mild or minor depression.

Traditional psychostimulants (amphetamine, methamphetamine, methylphenidate) improve energy, focus, and concentration. Individuals note these neurovegetative functioning inventory indices are dramatically impacted by depression, and respond quickly to psychostimulant medication. Often antidepressant medications will improve mood with lingering decrease in energy and focus. Adding a psychostimulant medication adjunctively enhances what the antidepressant doesn't complete. By improving energy, concentration, and focus, the individual is able to return to greater activity levels and "feels" better overall.

Thyroid stimulating therapies (synthroid, cytomel) are noted to increase energy and in the process improve mood. It is understood that a decrease in the function of the thyroid gland, hypothyroid function, results in fatigue, disrupted concentration, cold intolerance, and mood decrease. Synthroid is a synthetic form of T_4 and cytomel is a synthetic form of T_3. Each of these when taken orally augments and supplements the natural production of thyroid hormones by the thyroid gland. These thyroid hormones stimulate metabolism and other functions in the body to increase energy and enhance mood. When this augmentation approach is used, it is important to monitor serum TSH levels so as to maintain the individual within the appropriate reference ranges for TSH (0.4mIU/L to 4.0mIU/L). The dilemma is determining what an appropriate serum level is for a given individual. Individuals with no previous TSH level may appear "within normal limits", yet their thyroid gland may not be functioning to its appropriate level for them, and thus augmentation with either T_3 or T_4 may enhance their response to antidepressant medication by increasing metabolism and/or improving thyroid function.

Wellbutrin (bupropion) is often added to an SSRI either when the SSRI does not prove completely effective or when its benefit "poops" out. As bupropion is primarily dopaminergic, this improves focus, concentration, and energy. The dopamine also offsets weight gain and sexual dysfunction.

2. <u>The medication is effective and causes side effect(s)</u>. When an antidepressant medication proves effective in treating the mood disorder and has co-occurring side effects, the question arises as to changing the medication or adding another medication with it to offset the side effect(s) and maintain the antidepressant benefit. The most common side effects encountered secondary to the use of an SSRI antidepressant are:

   • Headache
   • Insomnia
   • Jitteriness
   • Sexual dysfunction
   • Stomach upset

   Typically the headache, insomnia, jitteriness and stomach upset resolve within 7 to 14 days. If they do not, it is prudent to change the medication. For insomnia, it is often a reasonable option to add in a medication to facilitate sleep if the antidepressant is showing good benefit for the depressive symptoms. Typically it is the sexual dysfunction side effect that persists. That can be improved by adding either Wellbutrin XL (bupropion hydrochloride) to the treatment regimen at 150mg, or by adding Viagra (sildenafil), Cialis (tadalafil), or Levitra (vardenafil). If none of these adjunctive approaches offsets the sexual dysfunction, then changing to another antidepressant medication is indicated.

3. <u>The medication is effective and then loses its effectiveness</u>. Some individuals report that after about two years of successful treatment with an SSRI, they experience a decrease in the effectiveness of the medication. The term for this is "SSRI poop-out." When this occurs there are 3 options:

   • Increase the dose of the current SSRI
   • Augment the SSRI with another medication
   • Change to another SSRI or other antidepressant family

   The first approach is to increase the dose, when possible. When augmenting, please refer to #1 above: atypical antipsychotic medications, Deplin (L-methylfolate), lithium, nontraditional stimulant medication (Provigil), traditional psychostimulants, thyroid stimulating therapies, and Wellbutrin XL.

4. <u>The disorder is part of a constellation of illnesses (comorbidities)</u>. If the medication is giving a modest amount of benefit yet not completely treating the individual, it is possible that the person has multiple comorbid illnesses and the antidepressant medication is treating specifically the depressive disorder. In this instance, it is important to add in other indicated medications that address the other specific medical/psychiatric disorder(s). Most common is the realization that the depressive disorder is actually a component of a bipolar disorder. When that is the case it is prudent to add a major mood stabilizer to the antidepressant medication. For many individuals depressive disorder will occur comorbidly with ADHD. Some individuals will suffer from Schizoaffective disorder in which case it is common to find the combination of an atypical antipsychotic and an antidepressant medication. While antidepressant medications help calm anxiety, it is noted that for some individuals an anti-anxiety medication may be necessary to add to the antidepressant as well.

APPENDIX 5

Overview of Psychotherapeutic Approaches

The following list is an overview of psychotherapeutic approaches with brief explanations:

- Behavior therapy is based upon operant conditioning and classical conditioning. This technique seeks to improve life function by rewarding beneficial behaviors and extinguishing destructive behaviors.

- Biofeedback is a technique that allows the individual to quantify his/her autonomic physiologic responses with his/her thoughts and to manage his/her thoughts to control his/her physiologic responses.

- Brief psychotherapy is an active and directive form of therapy or counseling that addresses life issues and stressors within a limited time frame of 20 sessions or less. Because of the limitation in time allowed for treatment, the therapist is more interventional with recommendations and feedback.

- Cognitive therapy is an approach developed by psychiatrist Aaron Beck in the 1960's. The concept is to identify and change distorted thought processes so as to improve behavioral and emotional responses.

- Cognitive Behavioral Therapy (CBT) is a combination of behavioral therapy and cognitive therapy that seeks to achieve change in the individual's life by recognizing both distorted thought processes and dysfunctional behaviors. These are improved by retraining thinking at the same time reinforcing positive behaviors and extinguishing negative behaviors.

- Crisis intervention is immediate short term assistance to guide an individual through an event that disrupts the individual's ability to cope. The goal is to assist the individual to return to pre-crisis life-skill function.

- Dialectical Behavior Therapy (DBT) is a therapy designed to help people change patterns of behavior that are not helpful, such as self-harm, suicidal thinking, and substance abuse. This approach works towards helping individuals increase their emotional and cognitive regulation. DBT is a modified form of cognitive-behavioral therapy that was developed in late 1970s by

Marsha M. Linehan to treat individuals with borderline personality disorder (BPD) and those with chronic suicidal ideations.

- Family therapy has at its core the goal of improving life functioning by recognizing the individual is part of a system (the family) and his/her actions affect every other member of the family system.

- Group psychotherapy has as its cornerstone the concept of individuals sharing their feelings while in a group and receiving support as well as thought provocation from others experiencing similar life issues. The group is directed by a trained therapist.

- Hypnotherapy is a technique whereby the therapist induces trance state in the individual seeking therapy, allowing the critical, analytical mind to dissociate, providing access to the feelings and thoughts stored in the unconscious mind. The purpose is to use the trance state as a tool to allow for the release of negative thoughts and the acceptance of healing suggestions. The ultimate goal is to ventilate the intrapsychic conflict and to harmonize the internal unconscious components of the mind.

- Marital therapy is a process whereby a couple with distress in their marriage works through the conflicts via the guidance of a therapist skilled in helping the partners come to understand themselves individually and the dynamics of the marital relationship based upon the issues each brings to the relationship.

- Psychoanalysis is the process developed by Sigmund Freud that allows the individual to verbalize thoughts and quantify feelings thereby revealing the unconscious conflicts that result in the symptoms and complaints bringing the individual into therapy. The role of the psychoanalyst is to guide the individual to a conscious understanding of these conflicts, allowing the individual to gain insight that results in the resolution of the unconscious intrapsychic conflicts.

- Psychodrama is a technique whereby individuals gain insight into their internal conflicts by acting them out with others in a choreographed play on stage under the direction of a therapist trained in this technique.

- Psychodynamic psychotherapy is similar to psychoanalysis in that the primary focus is to discover and uncover the individual's unconscious conflicts and gain insight, resolving the conflicts. The difference between this approach and psychoanalysis is that this form of therapy is less intensive both in time and approach, and allows for more interpersonal interaction by the therapist with the treated individual.

MEDICATION INDEX

INDEX

A

abstract, 111, 114, 194, 199, 201-202, 204
acetylcholine, 169-171
acne rosacea, 91
acute dystonic reaction, 40, 77-78
acute hepatotoxicity, 28
acute stress disorder, 9, 51-54, 124
addiction, 88
adjustment disorder, 9, 11-12, 54
adolescence, 32, 59, 71-72, 107-121, 125-126, 134
adrenal gland, 226
age-associated memory impairment, 166
agoraphobia, 9, 52, 55-59, 61-62, 126
agranulocytosis, 80, 229-230
AIMS, 85
akathisia, 21, 24, 40-41, 77-78, 80-81, 124, 150, 153-154, 168, 235
alcohol, 23, 57, 75, 87, 89, 91-94, 98, 100-101, 163-164, 178, 191-192, 204, 228, 238
alkaline phosphatase, 227, 229
Alzheimer, Alois, 168
Alzheimer's disease, 161, 164-165, 168-170, 172
amylase, 37, 229, 231
amyloid protein, 169
anal stage, 109
anergia, 16, 29, 35, 149
anhedonia, 13
anorexia, 113, 121, 128-131
anticholinergic, 21, 76, 78, 83, 163, 168
antidepressant, 16, 18-19, 21, 24, 26, 30-31
antisocial personality disorder, 101, 104, 106, 136
anxiety disorder, 51-55, 58-59, 61, 64-68, 117, 124, 126, 135, 137, 180, 195-196
anxious school refusal, 108, 123, 125-126
ascites, 92
Asher, Sir Richard, 187
Asperger's disorder, 107-108, 118-119
attention-deficit/hyperactivity disorder, 33, 88, 118, 133
atypical antipsychotic medications, 40-41, 43, 62, 66, 76, 79-85, 101, 140, 150, 163, 168, 230, 240, 243-246
atypical depression, 14-16, 29, 49-50
autistic disorder, 118-119
avoidant personality disorder, 105-106
axes, 189, 207-208

B

benign senescent forgetfulness, 166
Bennett, Abram E., 44
benzodiazepines, 41, 62-63, 66, 87, 89-90, 93, 128, 228
Bini, Lucio, 43
bipolar disorder, 9, 13, 31-47, 72, 74-75, 80-83, 98, 108, 135-136, 141, 149, 195, 203, 244, 247
Bleuler, Eugen, 72

Bleuler's 4 A's, 73
body dysmorphic disorder, 129, 183, 185
borderline personality disorder, 101, 104
brain abscesses, 162
Breuer, Joseph, 185
Briquet, Paul, 183
Briquet's syndrome, 183
bulimia, 128-131
BUN, 37, 229, 231

C

Cade, John F. J., 37
caffeinism, 57, 124
CAGE, 91
calcium, 81, 171-172, 229
cannabis sativa, 87, 228
cardiac ischemia, 162
catalepsy, 74
catatonia, 45-46, 72-73
catecholamine, 226
cerebral vascular accidents, 162, 223
Cerletti, Ugo, 43
Chase, Stella, 133
childhood, 32, 100, 107-109, 117-118, 133-134, 209
cholinergic blockade, 22
cholinesterase inhibitor, 170-172
cigarette, 87, 92, 94-95, 115, 149, 192
circadian rhythm, 134, 175-176, 238
cirrhosis, 92, 98
cluster A, 103, 106
cluster B, 104, 106
cluster C, 105-106
cocaine, 87, 192, 228
cognitive dulling, 39, 64, 82-83, 149
comorbidities, 30, 74, 135, 243, 246
compulsion, 60-61, 105
COMT, 20
concentration, 12-16, 29-30, 35, 47, 49-50, 54, 82, 118, 134, 138, 149, 153-155, 162, 164, 176, 180, 194-195, 219-221, 228, 245-246
conduct disorder, 83, 117, 135-136, 138-139, 154
confounders, 33, 135, 165
conscious, 9, 56, 97, 122, 126, 162-164, 183-188, 210, 213-223, 227, 250
continuous positive airway pressure, 174, 180
conversion disorder, 185, 210, 221
coprolalia, 139
copropraxia, 139
countertransference, 117, 208
cutters, 101
cyclothymic disorder (cyclothymia), 9, 41, 47,48, 72
cytochrome P450, 25, 27, 42, 148

D

DaCosta, Jacob Mendes, 51

defense mechanisms, 126, 137-138, 183-184, 187, 210, 215-216, 219-223, 241
delirium, 22, 45-46, 101, 161-164, 201, 203
delirium tremens, 93
delusional disorder, 9-10, 71-72, 74, 129, 183
delusions, 43, 71-75, 164, 168, 199, 204
dementia, 72, 101, 161-169, 186, 201, 203, 226-227
dementia praecox, 72
denial, 183, 216, 221
dependence, 31, 62-63, 88, 90-91, 117, 180
depolarization, 81, 171-172
depression, 11-37, 43-50, 64, 66-67, 74-75, 100, 108, 115, 128, 134, 164-165, 170, 221, 226, 230, 237, 239, 245
diabetes insipidus, 38, 122
diabetes mellitus, 41, 85 ,98, 122, 150, 207, 229
dietary interactions, 23, 67
discrete anxiety, 52, 55
displacement, 126, 216, 222
dopamine, 17,19-20, 24, 27, 29, 32, 40, 43, 50, 75-83, 88-89, 95, 101, 106, 115, 126, 140, 148, 150, 171, 181, 243, 246
dreams, 53-54, 218
Drug Enforcement Agency, 147
drug holiday, 158
Dupuytren's contractures, 92
dysdiadochokinesia, 84
dysthymic disorder, 9, 12
dystonic reaction, 40, 77-78, 150, 154, 235

E

early adolescence, 113-116, 126
eating disorders, 31, 71, 113, 117, 128-130
echolalia, 74
echopraxia, 74
ECT, 43, 46, 193
ego, 9, 109, 114, 123, 129, 134, 138, 161, 184, 198, 210, 213-216, 220-222
egocentric, 104, 109-110
electroconvulsive therapy, 43, 46, 193
elimination disorders, 117-120
encopresis, 117,120
enuresis, 31, 117, 120, 122-123, 230
Epworth Sleepiness Scale, 178
Erikson, Erik Homburg, 109, 111, 114
Esquirol, Jean Etienne, 59
euthymia, 11, 13, 47-48
excessive daytime sleepiness, 29, 88, 148, 173, 177, 179, 244
extrapyramidal side effects, 32, 40, 77-81

F

factitious disorder, 183, 186, 188
Falret, Jean Pierre, 72
fatigue, 29, 36, 59, 173-180, 219, 221, 228, 245
Fatigue Severity Scale, 179
first rank symptoms, 73
focal signs, 163
folie à deux, 74

folie circulaire, 72
formal stage, 111
Freud, Sigmund, 9, 51, 59, 108-111, 184-185, 196, 210-218, 220, 250,
frontal lobe release signs, 163

G

gamma-amino-butyric acid, 62, 94, 171, 238
gamma-glutamyltranspeptidase, 227
generalized anxiety disorder, 9, 25, 52, 58-59, 61, 64-67
genital stage, 110
GGT, 92,227
glaucoma, 39, 82, 149, 232
Global Assessment of Functioning, 207
glucose metabolism, 41, 59, 81, 85, 130, 150, 154, 161, 168, 176, 187, 225, 229-230
glutamate, 94, 171
Goldman Mood Map, 11
Goldman's Law of Medicine, 32
Goldman's reverse re-entry technique, 127
Goldman's rule of psychostimulants, 152
Goldman's theory of somatic consequences of repression, 221
Goldman's theory of status panicus, 56
grandiosity, 47
guilt, 13, 91, 111, 129, 216
gynecomastia, 80, 92

H

H$_2$ blockers, 82
hallucinations, 43, 71,73-75, 93-94, 101, 164, 168-169, 173-174, 186, 196, 199, 204, 226-227
hallucinogens, 75, 87, 192
Harrison act, 87
hebephrenia, 72
Hecker, Ewald, 72
hepatic encephalopathy, 37, 162, 227
heroin, 87, 228
Hirschsprung's disease, 120-121
histaminergic blockade, 22
histrionic personality disorder, 104, 106, 200, 207
human immunodeficiency virus, 178, 226
hyperactive child syndrome, 133
hypercholesterolemia, 151, 154, 168
hyperphagia, 16, 29, 49
hypersomnia, 16, 29, 49
hypertriglyceridemia, 151, 154, 168
hypnagogic, 173-174
hypnapompic, 174
hypnosis, 95, 121, 123, 209-210
hypnotics, 87
hypochondriasis, 185
hypoglycemia, 57, 163
hypomania, 11, 13 ,33-36, 47-48, 200, 203, 226
hypopnea syndrome, 29, 88, 138, 148, 173-174, 237, 244
hypotension, 23, 69, 129-130, 229
hypothermia, 129-130

projection, 216, 222
pseudodementia, 165
pseudologia fantastica, 186
psychoanalysis, 9, 184, 209-210, 250
psychostimulant, 75, 87-89, 136-141, 143, 145-148, 151-152, 154-155, 157-159, 180, 239, 243, 245-246
psychotherapy, 7, 43, 62, 69, 121, 131, 138, 207, 209-210, 212, 217, 220, 249-250
puberty, 110, 112-113

Q
QTc, 81

R
reaction formation, 216, 223
rebounding, 70, 136-137, 140-142, 150, 153, 238
repetitive transcranial magnetic stimulation, 46
repression, 110, 183, 216, 221
reuptake pump, 17, 21, 27, 29, 244
reverse re-entry technique, 127
role confusion, 112
rum fits, 93

S
SAMCEL(S), 14-15, 29, 34, 195-196
schizoaffective disorder, 9, 43, 75, 203, 247
schizoid personality disorder, 103, 106
schizophrenia, 9, 20, 40, 43-46, 72-75, 79-80, 95, 98, 108, 200, 209, 240
schizotypal personality disorder, 103, 106
Schneider, Kurt, 73
school phobia, 123-127
secondary gain, 183-184, 187
sedatives, 87, 239
self-injurious behavior, 101
sensorimotor stage, 110-111
separation anxiety, 60, 123-124, 126-127
sexual dysfunction 21, 23-25, 27-29, 67, 82, 246
shame, 13, 111, 129, 216-217
shift work sleep disorder, 29, 89, 139, 148, 174-175, 179-180, 237, 245
single photon emission computed tomography, 233
sleep deprivation, 174-176
sleep disorders, 29, 31, 89, 135, 138-139, 174-180, 196, 237, 245
social anxiety disorder, 25, 28, 53, 58-59, 64-68
social phobia, 9,52-53, 58-59, 61, 64-69
somatic triad, 183
somatization disorder, 185, 221
somatoform disorder, 183, 185, 188
specific phobias, 9, 52, 57-58
SSRI poop-out, 29, 32, 69, 246
SSRI, 21, 24-29, 32, 43, 50, 60-68, 70, 124, 128, 131, 143, 146, 246
status panicus, 56
Still, George Frederick, 133
sublimation, 216, 223
substance abuse, 31, 57, 75, 89, 117, 124, 135, 139, 191, 228

suicidal thoughts, 13-16, 34-35, 45, 49, 97-100, 104, 117, 152-155, 195-199
suicide, 34-35, 57, 89, 97-101, 196-197
sundowning, 162, 164-165, 170
superego, 9, 110, 113, 115-116, 161, 184, 210, 213-216, 220-221
Swedo, Susan E. ,60
syphilis, 191, 226

T
tangential thought, 199, 203
tardive dyskinesia, 40, 77-80, 84-86, 150, 154, 168, 235
testicular atrophy, 92
testosterone, 112-113
thought disorder, 9-10, 31, 37, 71, 75, 79-80, 83, 117, 131, 195-196, 200, 203-204, 209, 227, 237
thyroid function, 37-38, 42, 225-226, 231, 243, 245
tic disorders, 31, 117, 139, 198
tolerance, 62-63, 88, 90-91, 157, 239
Tourette's disorder, 108, 117, 131-132, 135, 139-140
toxic fumes, 163
transdermal, 23-24, 67, 95, 145-146, 154, 157-158
transference, 117, 208
treatment resistant, 44, 75
tremor, 40-41, 77, 79, 84-85, 93, 150, 154, 235
treponema pallidum, 226
tricyclic antidepressants, 21, 27, 62-63, 66, 88, 90, 127-128, 131, 146, 151-152, 168, 230
triglycerides, 41, 81, 85, 151, 154, 230
tryptophan, 20
tuberoinfundibular, 19, 80
typical antipsychotic medications, 76-80, 83-85, 132, 140
typical depression, 14-15
tyrosine, 19-20

U
unconscious, 9, 126, 137-138, 183-184, 186, 188, 210, 213-223, 241, 250

V
vagus nerve stimulation, 46
violent behavior, 97, 100
von Meduna, Ladislas J., 43
von Munchausen, Baron, 186-187
von Munchausen by proxy, 187
von Munchausen syndrome, 186

W
weight gain, 22-23, 25, 27-29, 38-40, 49-50, 70, 76, 80-82, 95, 131, 150, 159, 176, 240
Wernicke's encephalopathy, 92
Wernicke-Korsakoff syndrome, 92
Western blot, 226
Wolf-Parkinson-White syndrome, 52
worthlessness, 13

X
x-ray, 120, 163, 227,233-234

THE GOLDMAN GUIDE TO PSYCHIATRY
DSM-5 UPDATE
The Companion Guide

Effective 2013, the American Psychiatric Association published the DSM-5. This is the updated approach to diagnosis, a departure from the previous DSM-IV-TR. The DSM-IV-TR had provided a succinct, linear approach to diagnosis. The DSM-5 expands the diagnostic categories and groups them together in a broader method. The DSM-5 also provides for life-span disease identification.

GOLDMAN'S DIAGNOSTIC SCHEMA FOR THE DSM-5

MOOD DISORDERS	ANXIETY DISORDERS	THOUGHT DISORDERS

Bipolar and Related Disorders
• Bipolar I Disorder
  a) Manic Episode
  b) Hypomanic Episode
  c) Major Depressive Episode
• Bipolar II Disorder
  a) Hypomanic Episode
  b) Major Depressive Episode
	Anxiety Disorders
	• Agoraphobia
	• Generalized Anxiety Disorder
	• Panic Disorder
	• Selective Mutism
	• Separation Anxiety Disorder
	• Social Anxiety Disorder (Social Phobia)
	• Specific Phobia
		Schizophrenia Spectrum and Other Psychotic Disorders
		• Brief Psychotic Disorder
		• Delusional Disorder
		• Schizotypal (Personality) Disorder [criteria found in Personality Disorder section]
		• Schizoaffective Disorder
		• Schizophreniform Disorder
		• Schizophrenia

Depressive Disorders • Disruptive Mood Dysregulation Disorder • Major Depressive Disorder • Persistent Depressive Disorder [replacing DSM-IV-TR Dysthymic Disorder] • Premenstrual Dysphoric Disorder	**Obsessive-Compulsive and Related Disorders** • Body Dysmorphic Disorder • Excoriation (Skin Picking) Disorder • Hoarding Disorder • Obsessive-Compulsive Disorder • Trichotillomania (Hair Pulling Disorder)	
	Trauma and Stressor Related Disorders • Acute Stress Disorder • Adjustment Disorders • Disinhibited Social Engagement Disorder • Post-Traumatic Stress Disorder • Reactive Attachment Disorder	

The Goldman Guide to Psychiatry

A comparison of the tables of contents of both DSM guides gives a sense of the change via the "big picture":

DSM-IV-TR

Disorders Usually First Diagnosed in Infancy, Childhood, or Adolescence
Delirium, Dementia, and Amnestic and Other Cognitive Disorders
Mental Disorders Due to a General Medical Condition
Substance-Related Disorders
Schizophrenia and Other Psychotic Disorders
Mood Disorders
Anxiety Disorders
Somatoform Disorders
Factitious Disorders
Dissociative Disorders
Sexual and Gender Identity Disorders
Eating Disorders
Sleep Disorders
Impulse-Control Disorders Not Elsewhere Classified
Adjustment Disorders
Personality Disorders
Other Conditions That May Be a Focus of Clinical Attention

DSM-5

Neurodevelopmental Disorders
Schizophrenia Spectrum and Other Psychotic Disorders
Bipolar and Related Disorders
Depressive Disorders
Anxiety Disorders
Obsessive-Compulsive and Related Disorders
Trauma-and Stressor-Related Disorders
Dissociative Disorders
Somatic Symptom and Related Disorders
Feeding and Eating Disorders
Elimination Disorders
Sleep-Wake Disorders
Sexual Dysfunctions
Gender Dysphoria
Disruptive, Impulse-Control, and Conduct Disorders
Neurocognitive Disorders
Personality Disorders
Paraphilic Disorders
Other Mental Disorders
Medication-Induced Movement Disorders and Other Adverse Effects of Medication
Other Conditions That May Be a Focus of Clinical Attention

THE BIG PICTURE

The DSM-5 has modified the DSM-IV-TR in several ways. The DSM-5 approach discontinues the use of the 5-Axis diagnostic approach (the multi-axial approach). The DSM-IV-TR provided the clinician a schematic model with which to create a three-dimensional perspective of the patient, assessing the patient's acute psychiatric disorder, his/her intellectual capacity deficits and/or personality irregularities, his/her physical disabilities, his/her social distresses, and his/her numerical functioning scale via the multi-axial system. While the DSM-IV-TR utilized the clinician-subjective rating scale of the Global Assessment of Functioning [GAF] numerical scale, the DSM-5 has substituted the World Health Organization's WHODAS 2.0 assessment scale. The WHODAS scale is referenced to the ICD [International Classification of Disease] system. Many Government and Legal bodies still look to the DSM-IV-TR GAF scale when assessing disability.

The DSM-5 has modified the areas of Mood Disorders, Anxiety Disorders, and Thought Disorders. The Mood Disorders section has created new categories and modified DSM-IV-TR diagnoses. New specifiers have been added to the Mood Disorders section. So too, the Anxiety Disorders section has been modified to create three main categories, making Obsessive-Compulsive Disorder its own category. Also added as a new category is Trauma-and Stressor Related Disorders with 4 included Disorders. In the Thought Disorders category, Schizophrenia has become a spectrum, Delusional Disorder has removed the requirement of the delusions being NON-bizarre, and catatonia has been added as a specifier for mood disorders as well as psychotic disorders.

The DSM-5 has modified the section on intellectual capacity by removing "mental retardation" and changing the category to "Intellectual Disability" with severity being determined by adaptive functioning as opposed to IQ score [removing the term "retardation" is based on *Rosa's Law Public Law 111-256* signed into law October 5th, 2010].

The DSM-5 has consolidated Autistic Disorder and Asperger's Disorder into Autism Spectrum Disorder.

The DSM-5 has broadened Attention-Deficit/Hyperactivity Disorder to include criteria for Adult diagnosis.

The DSM-5 has deleted the 5 DSM-IV-TR subtypes of Schizophrenia. In the DSM-IV-TR if an individual experienced more than two voices conversing together, a single voice providing a running commentary of the patient's life, or suffered from bizarre delusions, either of those experiences would meet the initial criterion for a diagnosis of Schizophrenia. That has been changed to an individual requiring at least TWO symptoms from the criterion A section to be occurring and at least one of those must be either a fixed false belief (delusion), an auditory, visual, or tactile hallucination, or disorganized speech.

The DSM-5 has broadened the mood symptomatology for Schizoaffective Disorder to be present for the majority of the disorder's total duration.

MOOD DISORDERS [pages 11-50]

In the DSM-IV-TR, Mood Disorders tend to be linear and find themselves above or below the "usual and customary mood" designated as euthymia. Euthymia is mood that is not depressed, and not inappropriately elevated. Moods that drop below this "normal" mood equator are diagnosed in the DSM-IV-TR as an adjustment disorder, dysthymia, or major depressive disorder. Moods that rise above euthymia are hypomania or mania. Moods that go above euthymia AND below euthymia in the same person in alternating patterns are referred to as either cyclothymia (mild cycling moods) or bipolar disorder (with major swings in mood). In the DSM-IV-TR the concept of bereavement is not included in the mood disorders section, instead being coded as a V-code. In DSM-IV-TR, bereavement could give way to a Major Depressive Disorder if AFTER TWO MONTHS of grieving, the individual then demonstrated the criteria typically met for a major depressive episode.

DR. GOLDMAN'S MOOD MAP
Based on the DSM-IV-TR

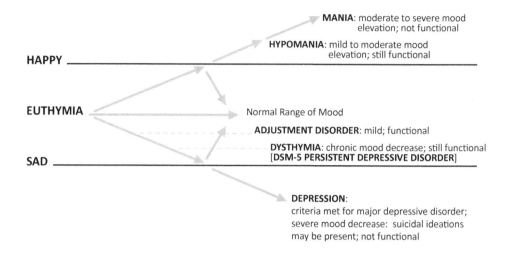

MANIA: moderate to severe mood elevation; not functional

HYPOMANIA: mild to moderate mood elevation; still functional

HAPPY

EUTHYMIA

Normal Range of Mood

ADJUSTMENT DISORDER: mild; functional

DYSTHYMIA: chronic mood decrease; still functional [DSM-5 PERSISTENT DEPRESSIVE DISORDER]

SAD

DEPRESSION:
criteria met for major depressive disorder; severe mood decrease: suicidal ideations may be present; not functional

GOLDMAN MOOD GUIDE
Based on the DSM-IV-TR

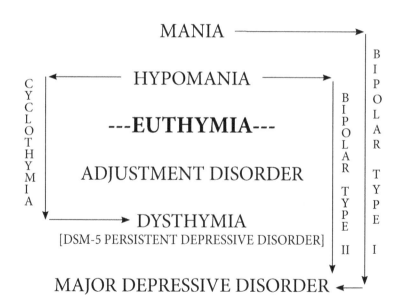

MANIA

HYPOMANIA

---EUTHYMIA---

ADJUSTMENT DISORDER

DYSTHYMIA
[DSM-5 PERSISTENT DEPRESSIVE DISORDER]

MAJOR DEPRESSIVE DISORDER

CYCLOTHYMIA

BIPOLAR TYPE II

BIPOLAR TYPE I

The DSM-5 has made changes from the DSM-IV-TR that expand and broaden the Mood Disorders Section:

A. Depressive Disorders
1) Two new categories have been added:
   a) Disruptive Mood Dysregulation Disorder
   b) Premenstrual Dysphoric Disorder
2) Dysthymic Disorder has been changed to: Persistent Depressive Disorder
3) Bereavement may have a co-occurring Major Depressive Episode and does NOT require the Bereavement to have lasted at least two months before being able to diagnose a depression.
4) There is a new modifier for Depressive Disorders: "with anxious distress"

B. Bipolar Disorders
1) For both hypomania and mania, along with changes in mood, there is an added emphasis on changes in activity and energy.
2) There is a new modifier for Bipolar Disorders: "with anxious distress"

Depressive Disorders

Disruptive Mood Dysregulation Disorder

This new category of disorder within the Mood Disorder Framework allows for characterizing and diagnosing children and adolescents with major mood disruption without labeling them with Bipolar Disorder prior to being 18 years of age.

In this disorder the hallmark is behavior [typically temper outbursts] that is out of proportion with the stimulating situation. The individual's verbal or physical outbursts are overdone in either intensity or duration, or both. To make this diagnosis, the individual must have had symptoms begin before the age of ten, the symptoms must have persisted for at least 12 months without a consecutive 3 month respite from symptoms, and the symptoms have to occur in at least 2 of the childhood 3-settings of home, school, and peer group. The individual must have an inter-ictal (period between temper outbursts) mood of irritability or anger that is observable by others most of the day, every day. The diagnosis is not made before the age of six or after the age of 18 years old. The diagnosis cannot co-occur with the diagnosis of Oppositional Defiant Disorder, Intermittent Explosive Disorder, or Bipolar Disorder.

Premenstrual Dysphoric Disorder

This new category of disorder within the Mood Disorder Framework recognizes serious disruption in mood and affect due to the monthly menstrual cycle. To meet the criteria for this diagnosis, the symptoms must be present in the week prior to the onset of menses, with symptom improvement within several days of the onset.

a) The patient must experience either mood swings, or marked irritability or anger, or feelings of depressed mood or hopelessness, or feelings of anxiousness.

b) The individual must also feel a disturbance in either sleep, appetite, concentration, or energy, or anhedonia, or a feeling of being overwhelmed, or physical discomfort of breast tenderness, or muscle pain, or subjective feelings of fluid retention or weight gain.

c) The individual must have had the above listed symptoms for most of her menstrual cycles for the past year.

Persistent Depressive Disorder [The DSM-5 Dysthymia]

The DSM-5 has combined chronic depression and dysthymic disorder into Persistent Depressive Disorder. In this disorder, the individual has experienced as in major depressive disorder of the DSM-IV-TR, depressed mood for most of the day every day, FOR AT LEAST 2 YEARS (in children and adolescents for at least one year). There must not have been a respite from symptoms for more than 2 months within this time frame. If the symptoms meet the standard criteria for a major depressive disorder, then this is a 2 year continuous major depression. If the symptoms traditional for a major depressive disorder are met, and instead the symptoms of only several neurovegetative functioning indices are met, then this is a dysthymic type of Persistent Depressive Disorder.

Per the DSM-5, if the individual meets the criteria for a Major Depressive Disorder for the required two week period, yet does not meet the 2 year period, then the diagnosis should be made as Major Depressive Disorder.

Bereavement [DSM-IV-TR versus DSM-5]

In the DSM-IV-TR there was a 2 month waiting period before grief and loss could be morphed into a diagnosis of Major Depressive Disorder. In the DSM-IV-TR it was felt that the loss of a loved one, the loss of physical health, personal belongings or other external issue, should not be given a Major Depressive Disorder diagnosis until after the 2-month period had passed and the individual demonstrated disturbance in the neurovegetative functioning inventories most of the day every day for at least two weeks, with the other important criteria being met of loss of interest in daily life activities (anhedonia), expressed feelings of depression, and/or the possible presence of suicidal ideations.

The DSM-5 has taken the perspective that one can slip into a Major Depressive Episode during the loss of a loved one, or other sense of grief and loss, if the individual experiences the usual and customary criteria for a Major Depressive Episode, even before the 2 months of grieving has passed. Hence the DSM-5 has deleted the DSM-IV-TR "exclusion" as it were. It is important to keep in mind that one can often distinguish grief from depression in that in grief:

    a) The decrease in mood typically comes in waves, instead of being most of the day every day;

    b) There is typically no loss of self-esteem in grief;

    c) The decrease in mood accompanying grief is thought appropriate and not "pathological" as in Major Depressive Disorder

Bipolar Disorders

In the DSM-IV-TR the hallmark of the Manic and Hypomanic components of Bipolar Disorder is the recognizable period of "abnormally and persistently elevated, expansive, or irritable mood" [page 169 DSM-IV-TR pocket desk reference ©2000 APA] whereas in the DSM-5 there is the addition of the increase in activity or energy required as well. The wording has been changed as follows:

"A distinct period of abnormally and persistently elevated, expansive, or irritable mood AND abnormally and persistently increased goal-directed activity or energy…" [page 65 DSM-5 pocket desk reference ©2013 APA].

While the DSM-IV-TR focused on mood with the clinician having an implicit understanding of the increase in activity and energy, the DSM-5 includes the focus on activity and energy in the precatory wording.

ANXIETY DISORDERS [pages 51-70]

The DSM-5 approach to Anxiety Disorders has modified the DSM-IV-TR approach from a single column of 9 main anxiety disorders [Panic Disorder Without Agoraphobia, Panic Disorder With Agoraphobia, Agoraphobia Without Panic Disorder, Specific Phobia, Social Phobia, Obsessive-Compulsive Disorder, Posttraumatic Stress Disorder, Acute Stress Disorder, Generalized Anxiety Disorder] to 3 columns divided into: Anxiety Disorders, Obsessive-Compulsive and Related Disorders, and Trauma- and Stressor-Related Disorders. The once all-inclusive Anxiety Disorder category has now released OCD, PTSD and ASD from its unidimensional classification and added Separation Anxiety Disorder and Selective Mutism.

The Anxiety Disorder column now includes:
- Separation Anxiety Disorder
- Selective Mutism
- Specific Phobia
- Social Anxiety Disorder
- Panic Disorder
- Agoraphobia
- Generalized Anxiety Disorder

The Obsessive-Compulsive and Related Disorders column includes:
- Obsessive-Compulsive Disorder
- Body Dysmorphic Disorder
- Hoarding Disorder
- Trichotillomania
- Excoriation Disorder

The Trauma- and Stressor-Related Disorders column includes:

- Reactive Attachment Disorder
- Disinhibited Social Engagement Disorder
- Posttraumatic Stress Disorder
- Acute Stress Disorder
- Adjustment Disorders [categorized by specifier: With depressed mood, With anxiety, With mixed anxiety and depressed mood, With disturbance of conduct, With mixed disturbance of emotions and conduct, Unspecified]

Anxiety Disorders

The DSM-5 has taken both Separation Anxiety Disorder and Selective Mutism from their original placement in the DSM-IV-TR chapter of Disorders Usually First Diagnosed in Infancy, Childhood, or Adolescence, and now placed them into Anxiety Disorders. The DSM-5 has dropped the requirement for symptoms of Separation Anxiety Disorder to have first occurred before the age of 18 years, and provides that in adults the symptoms must have persisted for at least 6 months. The core of Separation Anxiety Disorder is age inappropriate fear of being separated from an important attachment figure in the individual's life. The individual has to experience at least 3 of the following:

1) Physical symptoms at either the thought of being separated from the attachment figure or the actual occurrence
2) Excessive distress at the thought of being away from home or during the actual occurrence of being away from home
3) Excessive fear at the thought of losing the attachment figure, or harm coming to them
4) Excessive fear of something happening to the individual causing him/her to be away from their attachment figure
5) Reluctance or fear of leaving the home for fear of becoming separated from the attachment figure, such as going to school or work
6) Reluctance or fear to sleep away from the attachment figure
7) Reluctance and fear to be alone, without the attachment figure
8) Nightmares with the theme of separation

[pages 123-128]

The DSM-5 has placed the diagnosis of Selective Mutism into the Anxiety Disorder category, thus taking away the usual and customary classification of it being a childhood disorder. It requires a minimum of one month of consistently refraining from speaking in specific social situations where one is customarily expected to converse such as school or work. The individual does however converse freely in other settings, hence the issue of anxiety in the specified setting is the issue.

The DSM-5 has also disengaged Agoraphobia from Panic Disorder, so no longer is the diagnosis Panic Disorder With or Without Agoraphobia. Both Panic Disorder and Agoraphobia now stand alone as separate and distinct categories within Anxiety Disorders.

Obsessive-Compulsive and Related Disorders

The DSM-5 has expanded the concept of anxiety disorders into two new complete categories. The first expansion is spinning out OCD from the DSM-IV-TR Anxiety Disorder column. While OCD remains essentially the same, now into this category four other disorders have been added: Body Dysmorphic Disorder, Hoarding Disorder, Trichotillomania, and Excoriation Disorder. Body Dysmorphic Disorder was taken from the DSM-IV-TR Somatoform Disorders chapter and Trichotillomania was taken from the Impulse Control Disorders chapter. Hoarding Disorder and Excoriation (Picking) Disorders were DSM-IV-TR OCD subtypes that in DSM-5 have come of age into their own distinct diagnostic entities. [OCD pages 59-61]

Hoarding Disorder is a form of obsessive behavior hallmarked by the saving of items regardless of their inherent or intrinsic value. The individual has the obsessive need to save items and experiences distress/anxiety at the thought of discarding them. This typically results in the compromise of the use of one's living space [or work space] due to this over-accumulation of items. One's living space [or work space] becomes unmanageable unless there is intervention by a third party. Often as the individual develops an over-abundance of items within a given space, the internally perceived need to save the items for future use, results in the individual not being able to find what he/she is looking for due to the absolute clutter created.

Excoriation (Skin-Picking) Disorder is diagnosed when an individual engages in recurrent picking at one's skin, despite attempts to lessen or discontinue the behavior. As with all psychiatric disorders, it causes significant distress in the individual's life and/or social functioning.

Trichotillomania [Hair-Pulling Disorder] has been moved from the DSM-IV-TR category of Impulse-Control Disorders Not Elsewhere Classified to this section [Obsessive-Compulsive and Related Disorders] in the DSM-5.

Body Dysmorphic Disorder has been moved from the DSM-IV-TR category of Somatoform Disorders to this section [Obsessive-Compulsive and Related Disorders] in the DSM-5. In the DSM-5 the disorder is expanded to include a specifier regarding concerns about body muscular development. [pages 183-185]

The Trauma- and Stressor-Related Disorders

In the DSM-IV-TR, Acute Stress Disorder and Post-Traumatic Stress Disorder were both listed in the category of Anxiety Disorders. Reactive Attachment Disorder was listed and described in the category of Disorders Usually First Diagnosed in Infancy, Childhood or Adolescence. In the DSM-5, these psychiatric illnesses are now listed/described/diagnosed in this new category of Trauma- and Stressor-Related Disorders.

In DSM-IV-TR, Reactive Attachment Disorder served as the diagnosis and it had two types, either the Inhibited Type or the Disinhibited Type. In the DSM-5, Reactive Attachment Disorder has been modified to create two separate disorders:

1) Reactive Attachment Disorder
2) Disinhibited Social Engagement Disorder [which had essentially been the A2 criterion in the DSM-IV-TR Reactive Attachment Disorder description].

The essence of *Reactive Attachment Disorder* is the inability of the individual [beginning before age 5 years old] to establish close relationships with others, primarily caregivers, due to parental/caregiver disregard early on to the child's emotional and/or physical needs. The child manifests signs/

symptoms prior to the age of 5 years old. This is seen in neglectful homes of origin, and can be exacerbated by multiple foster placements wherein the child is unable to establish any close "parental" relationships.

The *Disinhibited Social Engagement Disorder* occurs in the child due to parental/caregiver disregard early on to the child's emotional and/or physical needs resulting in the child having no social/safety filter. This results in the child bonding to anyone and everyone who comes into his/her sphere of activity.

The DSM-5 has added greater depth and breadth to both Post-Traumatic Stress Disorder and Acute Stress Disorder. Unlike the DSM-IV-TR, both categories identify potential traumatic events as: "threatened death, serious injury, or sexual violence."

PTSD: The DSM-5 specifically notes criteria that apply to children above the age of 6 years old, adolescents, and adults. It then notes the criteria that apply for children 6 years old and younger. The essence is that the DSM-5 recognizes children as being PTSD sufferers, and it recognizes their symptoms are often different from the symptoms experienced by adults. [pages 54-55]

ASD: In the DSM-IV-TR duration must be at least two (2) days, whereas in the DSM-5 duration must be at least three (3) days. [pages 53-54]

The DSM-5 places **Adjustment Disorders** within this, the Trauma- and Stressor-Related Disorders category. The DSM-IV-TR had modifiers of Acute and Chronic, with Acute designating an adjustment disorder lasting less than 6 months and a Chronic adjustment disorder lasting more than 6 months. In the DSM-5, those modifiers are deleted, and it is merely noted that once the stressor is no longer present, the adjustment disorder should resolve within 6 months. [pages 11-12]

THOUGHT DISORDERS

Schizophrenia Spectrum and Other Psychotic Disorders [pages 71-86]

In the DSM-5 several psychiatric diagnoses are now listed in several categories, to wit, *Schizotypal (Personality) Disorder*. This diagnosis is found in both this section [Schizophrenia Spectrun and Other Psychotic Disorders] as well as in the Personality Disorders section. [pages 103-104]

Delusional Disorder in the DSM-5 no longer requires the circumscribed fixed-false belief (the delusion) to be non-bizarre. The key element is that other than related to the delusion, the individual's other behavior(s) is NOT bizarre or odd, and the individual's functioning is not disrupted other than related specifically to the circumscribed fixed-false belief(s). [page 71]

As in the DSM-IV-TR, the time frames for *Brief Psychotic Disorder* (1 day to 30 days), *Schizophreniform Disorder* (31 days to 6 months) and *Schizophrenia* (greater than 6 months) have remained the same. It is also of note that the DSM-5 has removed the concept of:

    a) Two or more voices conversing with each other, or
    b) A voice performing a running commentary of the patient's life, or
    c) A bizarre delusion

will alone suffice to meet the [A] criterion for making a diagnosis of *Schizophrenia*. The DSM-5 now requires at least two (2) of the following and at least one (1) of the two must come from the first three (3) listed symptoms:

    a) Delusions
    b) Hallucinations
    c) Disorganized speech
    d) Grossly disorganized behavior
    e) Negative symptoms (apathy, alogia, anergy)

The DSM-IV-TR listed five (5) sub-types of Schizophrenia [Paranoid type, Disorganized type, Catatonic type, Undifferentiated type, and Residual type]. The DSM-5 has discarded the five (5) sub-types. [pages 72-75]

DSM-5 NEW CATEGORIES

Somatic Symptom and Related Disorders
[pages 183-188]

The DSM-5 created new category divisions and has discarded the following disorders:

a) Somatization Disorder [pages 185-186]
b) Hypochondriasis [page 185]
c) Pain Disorder [page 185]

The DSM-5 has moved Body Dysmorphic Disorder from Somatoform Disorders to: Obsessive-Compulsive and Related Disorders

The new DSM-5 Category is Somatic Symptom and Related Disorders [Somatoform Disorders in DSM-IV-TR]. Found within this grouping are:

a) *Somatic Symptom Disorder*: one or more somatic complaints that are disruptive to the person's life, typically persist(s) more than 6 months in duration, and may have pain as its predominant complaint.

b) *Illness Anxiety Disorder*: As the name implies, the individual has a preoccupation with the possibility of having or developing an illness. This preoccupation has persisted for more than 6 months. The individual regularly assesses self for the possibility of illness. If the individual does have somatic symptoms, they are mild at most. This generates a large amount of anxiety for the individual.

c) *Conversion Disorder*: The individual has an alteration or decrement in voluntary motor function or neurological function that does not have a true underlying medical or neurological cause. Acute presentation is less than 6 months and persistent presentation is greater than 6 months. [page 185]

d) *Psychological Factors* Affecting Other Medical Conditions: The individual has an actual medical condition that is negatively impacted by psychological or behavioral issues.

e) *Factitious Disorders*:
   i- Imposed on self [DSM-IV-TR Munchausen's] the individual creates signs/symptoms of an underlying physical or mental illness or injury. This behavior occurs even if no demonstrable gain is evident. [pages 183-188]

ii- Imposed on Another (person) [DSM-IV-TR Munchausen's by Proxy] the individual creates symptoms of an underlying physical or mental illness or injury in another person (the proxy). This behavior occurs even if no demonstrable gain is evident. [page 187]

The DSM-IV-TR presented Attention-Deficit/Hyperactivity Disorder along with Oppositional Defiant Disorder and Conduct Disorder as independent discrete categories in the section Disorders Usually First Diagnosed in Infancy, Childhood or Adolescence, while presenting them as a continuum progression of behavioral disorder. Also in this section were Asperger's Disorder and Autistic Disorder as discrete diagnoses while presenting a continuum as well. Found within this category were the communication disorders, hence tying them all together. The DSM-5 focuses on neurodevelopment and includes intellectual capacity disability [replacing the term mental retardation] with Autism, ADHD, Learning Disorders, Communication Disorders, and Motor Disorders. The DSM-5 has deleted the distinct category of Asperger's Disorder, instead providing a scale of disruption as level one through three in the Autism Spectrum Disorder. Oppositional Defiant Disorder and Conduct Disorder have been removed from this section and placed into Disruptive, Impulse-Control, and Conduct Disorders [which also includes Antisocial Personality Disorder, hence creating a new behavioral continuum without ADHD being at the front of the progression.]

Neurodevelopmental Disorders

1) As noted earlier, the term mental retardation has been deleted from DSM-5, and in its place is the term *Intellectual Disability (Intellectual Developmental Disorder)*. Severity of the disability is no longer determined specifically by IQ scores, instead it is determined by adaptive functioning.

2) In DSM-5 *Autism Spectrum Disorder* has at its core two components
   a) Deficits in social communication and social interaction, and
   b) The presence of restricted-repetitive behaviors, interests, and activities [pages 118-119]

3) *Attention-Deficit/Hyperactivity Disorder* in DSM-5 has been expanded to include criterion items that allow for ADHD to have application across the life-span into adulthood. The age before which ADHD is diagnosed has been increased from symptoms prior to age seven years old to "several inattentive or hyperactive-impulsive symptoms" being present prior to the age of twelve years old. The diagnostic criteria now specify individuals 17 years of age and older, and the traditional criteria of 6 or more is lessened to 5 or more for adults. [pages 133-136]

4) *Tic Disorders and Tourette's Disorder* are moved into this DSM-5 category under the subheading of Motor Disorders, from the DSM-IV-TR category of Disorders Usually First Diagnosed in Infancy, Childhood or Adolescence. [pages 139-140]

Disruptive, Impulse-Control, and Conduct Disorders

As noted above, Intermittent Explosive Disorder, Oppositional Defiant Disorder, Conduct Disorder, and Antisocial Personality Disorder [still also listed in the Personality Disorder section] are now placed into this category. This creates an "angry" behavior continuum with a disregard for others. Each of these disorders is essentially the same as found in the DSM-IV-TR, except Oppositional Defiant Disorder in the DSM-5 is given greater definition. *Oppositional Defiant Disorder* is fleshed out with internal components of:

a) Angry/Irritable Mood
b) Argumentative/Defiant Behavior
c) Vindictiveness [added new; not specified in DSM-IV-TR] [pages 136-137]

Neurocognitive Disorders

The DSM-IV-TR chapter Delirium, Dementia, and Amnestic and Other Cognitive Disorders has been replaced by this new DSM-5 designation. This new DSM-5 chapter discusses minor and major neurocognitive deficits and utilizes the different types of dementing illnesses as the specifiers. In a way this is at one end of the life-span continuum of Neurodevelopmental Disorders to Neurocognitive Disorders.

This book serves as the guide to the transition from the DSM-IV-TR to the DSM-5 initially identifying the broad modifications and changes from the one to the other. The DSM-5 is still in flux and is still not fully incorporated into all practices as of early 2016. The ICD-10 is the International Statistical Classification of Diseases and Related Health Problems (ICD) compiled by the World Health Organization to provide coding for signs, symptoms, and diseases. The current code numbers found in the ICD-9 are currently transitioning to the ICD-10 effective October of 2015. The DSM-5 was formulated to correspond to the ICD-9/10.

* * * * *

The page numbers found within this text in brackets [example: pages x-x+1] correspond to the DSM-IV-TR sections in *The Goldman Guide To Psychiatry*. This new book in combination with *The Goldman Guide To Psychiatry* and *The Goldman Guide To Psychiatry Review Guide*, serves for classroom study, Board Exams, use in rotations, and for use in clinical practice. Videos of Dr. Goldman's lectures and DVD's on Psychiatry as well as Medical Jurisprudence/Medical Ethics can be ordered online from Amazon. These may also be accessed via www.thegoldmangroup.org

Updated Antidepressants

Fetzima (milnacipran): inhibits norepinephrine and serotonin reuptake. It is touted to treat focus, function, and fatigue. FDA-approved July 26th, 2013.

Trintellix (vortioxetine): selectively inhibits serotonin reuptake; antagonizes serotonin 5-HT3 receptors; agonizes serotonin 5-HT1A receptors. Due to potential initial gastro-intestinal upset or headache, it is best initiated as 5mg orally at bedtime for at least 5 nights, then it can be changed to morning dosing and may be increased to 10mg after the first 5 days. FDA-approved as Brintellix (vortioxetine) to treat major depressive disorder September 30th, 2013. On May 2nd, 2016, it was renamed Trintellix (vortioxetine) in the United States to avoid name confusion with the blood-thinning medicine Brilinta (ticagrelor).

Viibryd (vilazodone): selectively inhibits serotonin reuptake and partially agonizes serotonin 5-HT1A receptors. It should be taken with 350 calories of food. FDA-approved January 24th, 2011 to treat major depression; Actavis received FDA-approval for once daily dosing as 20mg March 16th, 2015.

Updated Atypical Antipsychotics

Latuda (lurasidone): antagonizes dopamine D2 receptors and serotonin 5-HT2A receptors. It should be taken with 350 calories of food to provide for its full absorption. Failure to take with food can result in on 30% to 50% absorption of the medication. FDA-approval for Latuda (lurasidone) for schizophrenia occurred October 28th, 2010. On July 1st, 2013, the FDA approved Latuda (lurasidone) for monotherapy and adjunctive therapy in adult patients with bipolar depression. On January 28th, 2017, the FDA approved Latuda (lurasidone) for treating adolescent schizophrenia in ages 13 years to 17 years old.

Rexulti (brexpiprazole): partially agonizes dopamine D2 and serotonin 5-HT1A receptors; antagonizes serotonin 5-HT2A receptors. FDA-approved for treating schizophrenia and adjunctive treatment for major depressive disorder July 10th, 2015. The FDA approved its use for maintenance treatment for schizophrenia September 23rd, 2016.

Saphris (asenapine): antagonizes dopamine D2 receptors, serotonin 5-HT2A receptors. Saphris (asenapine) is not taken as a traditional oral medication. Instead it is used either sublingually (under the tongue) or placed into the cheek. It then dissolves and results in oral-buccal mucosal absorption. It is believed to deliver a more rapid onset of benefit due to this form of delivery. For best effectiveness, one should not eat or drink for 10 minutes prior to taking or for 10 minutes after taking the medication. Saphris (asenapine) received its FDA-approval for use September 7th, 2010. March 13th, 2015, it received FDA approval for pediatric use 10 years of age and older for bipolar I disorder.

Vraylar (cariprazine): partially agonizes dopamine D2, dopamine D3, and serotonin 5-HT1A receptors; it antagonizes serotonin 5-HT2A receptors. It has greater affinity for dopamine D3. It is thought to have cognitive enhancing qualities. Vraylar (cariprazine) received FDA approval for treating schizophrenia and bipolar disorder in adults effective September 17th, 2015.

NEW MEDICATION UPDATE
INDEX

DSM-5 COMPANION UPDATE INDEX

51778506R00154

Made in the USA
Columbia, SC
23 February 2019